LIVE
OR
DIE

Thomas H. Ainsworth, M.D.

LIVE
OR
DIE

MACMILLAN PUBLISHING COMPANY

New York

Reprinted by permission of *New England Journal of Medicine*, 296:601, 1977: Breslow, L. and Somers, A. "Lifetime Health Monitoring Program." Excerpts from this article appear in Chapter 23.

Macmillan Publishing Company
866 Third Avenue, New York, N.Y. 10022
Collier Macmillan Canada, Inc.

Library of Congress Cataloging in Publication Data

Ainsworth, Thomas H.
Live or die.
Bibliography: p.
1. Medicine—United States.   2. Medical care—
United States.   3. Medicine, Preventive—United States.
I. Title.
R151.A36   1983   362.1'0973   83-870
ISBN 0-02-500640-1

10 9 8 7 6 5 4 3 2 1

Designed by Jack Meserole

Printed in the United States of America

FOR Sandy,

MY WIFE AND BEST FRIEND

FOR THIRTY-THREE YEARS

Each age is a dream that is dying
or one that is coming to birth.

—FRANKLIN DELANO ROOSEVELT

CONTENTS

Contents

PART TWO   How to Reclaim Your Own Life

Contents

INTRODUCTION

I am a physician, and this book is about my profession. More precisely, it's about the way medicine is practiced in the United States today.

I'm concerned about the direction medicine has taken and I'm frightened about its future. Make no mistake, we have the best system of illness care the world has ever seen. But we have to ask some serious questions: Why does the system ignore the health of those it claims to be serving? And at a time when we are capable of preventing at least half of all diseases we encounter, why are we spending nearly all our money and effort on the *treatment* of illness and only a pittance on its *prevention*? (We could, right now, be preventing 90% of the big killers—heart disease, lung cancer, and stroke—which account for 70% of all deaths and disabilities.)

The answers to these questions are intimately entangled in the root causes of the greatest problem we are struggling with today—the rapidly escalating cost of medical care. Given enough time, we might have been able to straighten out, one-by-one, some of the causes of high cost: the perverse incentives built into the way we pay doctors and hospitals, overspecialization by physicians, and lack of planning, which produced an oversized system that is providing much more care than we need—just to pay its rent.

But we have run out of time. High cost is no longer simply a problem for the individual consumer; it is now interfering with the priorities of business, labor, and government to a troublesome degree. And all three are demanding that the system be overhauled immediately, before it bankrupts us.

High cost has created a true dilemma and none of the solutions currently being proposed are desirable or acceptable. Nevertheless, government is taking actions almost daily that could radically change the way medical care is provided. Tenets we have long held dear, such as the freedom of choice of our physician, are in danger of being sacrificed in order to contain costs. We are fast approaching the point where we could be witnessing a preposterous paradox—the rationing of medical care, not because of a shortage of care, but because we are providing too much care.

Most Americans are unaware of how changes now being proposed will determine the kind of medical care they will receive in the future, or how these changes could affect their health and their pocketbooks. Some will support any change because of a growing disenchantment with the present system, prompted not only by high costs but by what appears to be a lack of caring on the part of the physician. Some are turning to alternative therapists, cultists, and faddists—who may actually prove to be hazardous to their health—for needs that the medical profession seems to regard as unimportant. Others continue to have blind faith in the Medical Establishment and fail to take any personal responsibility for their own health. They all need to realize that only when they become informed consumers will they be able to demand a health care system that truly meets their needs.

Many physicians are seemingly unaware as the medical consumer that there is anything wrong with the present system and so fail to see that change is necessary and inevitable. Others are hostile to any suggestion that could disrupt the status quo, where they feel most comfortable. I know from experience how easy it is to become so involved in your own practice that your view of the overall system becomes myopic. It wasn't until I entered the field of administrative medicine, after twenty years of private practice, that I was able to see flaws in the system that had previously seemed so perfect to me. By joining the higher echelons of the Medical Establishment, I had the opportunity to examine it; I saw how it worked, listened to its heart, lived with it. And now I know I must write about it.

This book is an urgent appeal to the members of my profession to face honestly the problems besetting the system and to take a leadership role in bringing about the changes that will assure affordable health care which retains the many excellent aspects of our present system—especially its freedom—and yet is tailored to the real needs of the American people.

The book is also a love story about my love for my profession; I hope this feeling comes through, even though I call attention to its faults, as one might do concerning a wayward child who in many ways is irresponsible and, consequently, not achieving an easily reached potential.

In addition, the book is a romance about the affair my profession has been having with technology. Its seduction has been easy, because there seems to be a technical solution to every problem. The affair has been a heady one, enough to make some physicians think they can play God. And when you're up there in the clouds, how can you be bothered with such mundane concerns as the cost of medical care? "We're able to transplant hearts," they shout, "and you're worried about how much it costs?"

The ending to the affair hasn't been written. The liaison between medicine and technology continues; but I think there could be a happy ending. I hope so. I care.

Carmel Valley, California
January 1983

A Matter of Life
and Death

It's a matter of life and death. It affects us all. Yet most of us are not aware that our lives are endangered by something we least suspect and most trust—the contemporary medical care system.

We have developed an almost religious faith in this system, in what I call the Medical Establishment. We have abdicated responsibility for our own lives and look to an authority, a father figure, to ensure our good health. Our faith in this authority is now so great that we believe we can eat, drink, and be merry without thought for the morrow, because, if we become ill, we are certain the Medical Establishment will come rushing to save us with the latest miracle cure.

Don't count on it. Usually it is too late and the miracle cure is too often more—or less—than we bargained for. Take the case of Adam Americus.

◄§ Adam, who was born in 1930, was a child of the Depression, a teenager during World War II, an all-American football player in college. He was drafted into the army after graduation and spent two years in Korea. When he took off his army uniform, he easily slipped into the male middle-class harness. He married his childhood sweetheart and became a father and an M.B.A. a year later. He went to work for one of the "big eight" accounting firms and learned how to work under pressure to meet deadlines, solving other people's problems. He thrived on competition and rapidly fought his way from consultant to manager to partner in five years. He sired three more children at two-year intervals and then had a vasectomy on the advice of his wife's obstetrician.

Recently, Adam had an affair with his secretary that has cinched his harness even tighter. As penance, he is working harder and has started going to church on Sunday. He eats more, smokes more, drinks more. The competition is getting tougher and his indigestion more frequent. He buys Tums by the gross.

1

Adam approaches his annual physical, which his firm insists on, with typical macho bravado. He has always denied any real symptoms. Each year he receives the same casual warnings and advice from the company doctor. "Your blood pressure is a little high and your cholesterol is up a bit. You should take more time off, relax more, lose some weight, and cut down on your smoking," the doctor says, as he pats his own paunch and blows smoke in Adam's face.

In 1975, at the age of forty-five, Adam has a coronary, which sidelines him for the first time since an ankle sprain during his sophomore year in college. He is furious. As soon as he is out of the coronary intensive care unit, he begins smoking again. As soon as he gets home, he resumes his evening cocktails. He is back at work three weeks later. He does agree to take the medication prescribed for his high blood pressure, but he soon gives that up when he realizes it's causing him to become impotent. "Damn it," he yells at the doctor, "if I can't get a hard-on, my blood pressure will go through the ceiling."

"Okay, okay," the doctor soothes him.

Two years later Adam has a second coronary. It happens at the lunch table when he is dining with his boss and their most important client. If it weren't for the paramedics in the fire department ambulance, Adam would be a statistic—one of the 60% of coronary occlusion victims who die before they reach the hospital. But the paramedics keep him breathing with mouth-to-mouth resuscitation and his heart pumping with external cardiac massage until they arrive at the emergency room, where the fibrillation (or quivering) of his heart muscle is interrupted with electric shock. His heart starts beating again on its own.

"You're a young man, Adam," begins the cardiac surgeon, who is consulted four weeks later.

You look pretty young yourself, thinks Adam.

"You're fortunate that we have a new operation that will revascularize your heart."

He looks like an all-American. I wonder where he played football.

"We simply bypass that right coronary artery of yours that got plugged up and caused this heart attack."

He can't be much over thirty. I wonder who he is.

"You had a very bad attack this time. You knocked out one artery completely. The angiogram today showed you have pretty extensive coronary disease."

Angiogram? "Oh, yes," Adam says. He remembers the word from his previous hospitalization. A special procedure, the nurse in X ray said as she gave him a shot. He remembers his groin being washed with something cold that ran down, burning his scrotum. He remembers the flush that kept getting hotter until he thought his head would explode, and then the pain in his chest. After that he must have passed out. Angiogram. "Oh, yes," he says. "X rays of my coronary arteries."

"You don't want to be a cardiac cripple at your age. You're a dynamic, hardworking man, and your family depends on you."

Family depends on me, thinks Adam.

"If you say the word we can go ahead in the morning. There is time on the schedule."

Family depends . . . morning . . . schedule . . . angiogram. "Oh, yes," he says.

The doctor has made the decision. It is too late for Adam to take responsibility for his own life, and his wife shares his faith in the Medical Establishment.

Adam has a third coronary occlusion the following morning, during the course of his bypass surgery. Once again, he survives. ∂●

The year 1977 was a very good year for aortocoronary bypass grafting, the official name of the procedure—a $1.5 billion year. The operation was performed 70,000 times in the United States. The average hospital bill for each procedure was $12,500 and, while nobody will confirm it, in many cases the surgeon's fee approached $10,000.

Adam was lucky. In the university hospital where he was operated on, 1977 marked the tenth year that bypass surgery had been performed. The mortality rate had been reduced gradually from 10% in 1968 to 1.7%. Now everyone was happy; the acceptable mortality rate of 1% for elective procedures was well in sight. Only 26 out of 1,517 cases had died that year; Adam was a survivor.

Adam's cousin was not so lucky. He had the same procedure done in a community hospital where only three bypass operations were performed in 1977. Before Adam's cousin was operated on, the mortality rate for bypass surgery in that hospital had been zero; after his surgery it was 33%. Everyone blamed Adam's cousin for ruining their statistics; he had chosen the wrong hospital.

In a month, Adam is feeling great. He has no symptoms and can't wait to get back into his harness. The cardiac surgeon is as pleased as Adam is with the result of the operation, and he raises his fee 10% to keep up with the rising cost of living for the lifestyle to which he has recently become accustomed. But he neglects to warn Adam that the operation is still experimental and is designed only to relieve intractable angina, the disabling pain that does not respond to good medical management and medication. He does not tell him that the operation has not affected the underlying cause of his heart attack: the disease called atherosclerosis that is continuing to harden his coronary arteries. Furthermore, he neglects to tell Adam that the relief of the mild symptoms of angina he has had as a result of the surgery may give him a false sense of security, as he probably will not experience severe angina —the chest pain that occurs on exertion and is the body's warning signal that the heart is being overtaxed. る

Had aortocoronary bypass grafting (ACBG) been a new drug instead of a new operation, the Federal Drug Administration (affectionately referred to by the Medical Establishment as "that damned FDA") would have insisted on a package insert warning of side effects and potential dangers to the patient. But where do you insert a warning about a new operation? Certainly not in the envelope with the bill, and it would be malpractice to leave it in the wound.

If there were such a warning, it might read something like this:

Once aortocoronary bypass grafting is performed, medical therapy must remain an essential component of management, the goal being normal blood pressure, total abstinence from smoking, achievement of the lowest possible lipid levels, and adherence to ideal body weight and principles of physical conditioning. Because ACBG does not reverse the basic pathologic process of atherosclerotic occlusive disease it represents at best a new lease on life which is temporary. If ACBG is to offer anything more than a partial reprieve or a stay of execution in patients with coronary artery disease, serious medical management must be undertaken with the aim of reversing, or at least arresting, the underlying disease process.*

In essence, once you get around the medicalese, this warning translates simply:

Just because you have had an operation, don't think you have been cured. The operation was designed to relieve only the symptoms of intractable angina. Your symptoms are gone, but you still have the underlying disease, which continues to cause hardening of your coronary arteries. If you are serious about stopping the continuing degenerative process of the disease, you must follow a strict medical regimen that you should have adopted before you had your operation. You must maintain normal blood pressure, preferably by using

* These words were taken from an article on aortocoronary bypass grafting: Aortocoronary Bypass Grafting in the Management of Patients with Coronary Artery Disease by Robert A. Boccino and Henry D. McIntosh.

N.B.: See Bibliography for complete publication data for all articles and books cited in footnotes.

modern behavior modification techniques for stress management (your doctor should be able to tell you how to do this) or through medication (your doctor knows all about this). You must abstain totally from the use of tobacco—this includes pipes, cigars, and chewing tobacco, as well as cigarettes. You must eat foods that will keep the lipids (fatlike substances) such as cholesterol, triglycerides, and low-density lipoproteins at lower than normal levels in your blood (your doctor should be able to tell you how to do this without medication). You should balance your food intake and exercise to maintain your normal weight. You should stay in good general physical condition by doing regular aerobic exercises supervised by your doctor. *Do not go out and jog without first consulting your doctor!*

But no one warned Adam. He went back to his high-pressure job, his smoking, his overeating, his alcohol, his family, and his new secretary. He never felt better in his life. His faith in the Medical Establishment had never been greater.

The Medical Establishment, furthermore, had never had greater faith in an operation. That the bypass operation was an answer to the disabling effects of intractable angina and markedly improved the quality of life for angina sufferers was not the only basis for this faith. The Establishment, whose acute vision rarely loses sight of profits on the horizon, sustained its faith on the *hope* that the operation would also prove to prolong life and decrease the frequency of subsequent heart attacks.

At no time, however, has there been objective supporting evidence to justify this hope. Nevertheless, an increasing number of patients without intractable angina have undergone bypass surgery as a preventive procedure despite the lack of evidence to support the operation's effectiveness for anything more than relief of angina symptoms.

Most of these operations have been performed as controlled clinical trials, an ethical form of human experimentation, to determine whether or not the operation will prove to do everything the Medical Establishment hopes it will. A great deal is riding on the demonstration of this proof because if medical evidence supports the *hope* that the operation prolongs life and decreases the occurrence of heart attacks, the Establishment's annual income will escalate by many billions of dollars.

Doctors could then routinely order angiograms for millions of asymptomatic or mildly symptomatic persons at high risk of having coronary artery disease, hundreds of thousands of whom will show some evidence of atherosclerosis. Armed with this supporting data, bypass grafting can then be justified for vast numbers of people without angina symptoms. You can see why the Establishment couldn't wait until the results of the controlled clinical trials were reported.

And they haven't waited. Perhaps this is because the Medical Establishment is so far above the rest of us that it can see beyond the horizon. Apparently they can see a time when anyone with coronary artery disease can demand a bypass operation to prevent the first coronary occlusion. This prediction is not extreme. The publication of a survey of cardiac surgeons who believe this will occur, precipitated an editorial by E. Braunwald in a 1977 issue of the *New England Journal of Medicine* that cautioned surgeons about the ethical and socioeconomic implications of extending and expanding the use of bypass operations to patients for whom the indications were not clearly established.

The cost of such a prospect is mind-boggling. Using 1979 data, if the then-prevalent coronary artery disease population of 4,600,000 is multiplied by a hospital bill of $12,500, the cost of using this surgery as a preventive measure for those afflicted with coronary heart disease is a staggering total of $57.5 billion—or 27% of the total U.S. health care budget for that year.

Whether it is faith, hope, or charity that motivates cardiac surgeons (with whom, it has been reported, God talks directly) is irrelevant; they are tooling up for the official acceptance of this miraculous breakthrough —miraculous because it comes just in time to save the cardiac surgery industry from bankruptcy. This industry expanded and flourished after another breakthrough—open heart surgery, which made it possible to correct nearly all congenital heart defects. But all too soon, the defects had been corrected and there was no backlog. There was a glut of cardiac surgeons on the market and they began to have nightmares of driving taxicabs. Then along comes the bypass operation, and, instead of mothballing cardiac surgery suites, hospitals are expanding them. Even community hospitals that do no other cardiac surgery are preparing to do the bypass operation.

Surgical suites are only the beginning. A hospital-based industry has also been created to support the surgery. Cardiac catheterization labs with X-ray facilities for angiograms, heart-lung machines, monitoring equipment, and coronary intensive care units are all necessary adjuncts. A cadre of technicians and nurse-specialists is also necessary to support the surgical team. Coronary bypass surgery, unknown fifteen years ago, is now a $3.3-billion-a-year industry. How's that for a miracle?

Adam was a victim of this miracle. He died of his fourth coronary in 1980 at the age of fifty. He spent the last three weeks of his life in a coronary intensive care unit, where he had three cardiac arrests and three successful resuscitations. His brain died during the last resuscitation, but no one had the courage (or the honesty) to discontinue the life-support systems until three days later, when his hospital bill hit $30,000.

This must be said of Adam Americus: He participated and paid his own way in the biggest and best experiment the Medical Establishment has ever conducted. The results of the clinical trials were made available in 1978. Adam helped prove, as the results of the clinical trials report, that the aortocoronary bypass grafting procedure is of no value in reducing mortality, decreasing the frequency of subsequent heart attacks, or increasing the longevity of patients with coronary artery disease. Its only proven indication is to relieve the pain of intractable angina. (There is some evidence, however, that it may also prevent premature death in a limited number of patients with angina who have a complete block of the left main coronary artery.)

Nevertheless, the faith of the Medical Establishment lives on. Clinical trials continue, but they are no longer controlled. "It's a different operation today than it was five years ago," claim the cardiac surgeons. "It would be unfair to judge the procedure on what we were doing then." They still hope for a different result. They want the operation to do what they think it should do, and so they are trying harder. They now perform 165,000 bypass operations a year at a cost of $20,000 each. That the average annual income of the 700 cardiac surgeons who perform most of these operations exceeds $1 million is not the primary incentive. Cardiac surgeons are having a love affair with technology.

The greatest tragedy in Adam's case is not that he did not have intractable angina and, therefore, had an unnecessary operation (adequate medical management could have given him the same, if not greater, chance for survival). The tragedy is that he could have avoided coronary artery disease in the first place. The medical profession has been so engrossed in treatment that it has lost interest in preventing disease. If the physician who performed Adam's annual physical had put him on a strict medical regimen, the same regimen he should have been placed on following his surgery, he probably would never have suffered a coronary occlusion.

Adam never took responsibility for his own health. After he recovered from his first coronary he was unable to reclaim his own life because he had neither the cooperation of the Medical Establishment nor an adequate knowledge of what he could do on his own.

This book could have saved Adam's life. It could have provided him with the knowledge necessary to confront life, not death. From the first part of this book, he would have gained insight into the Medical Establishment. He would have learned how and why it operates as it does. When he needed to, he would have known how to deal with the Establishment in partnership with his physician—as an equal, a client, not in the traditional obsequious role of the passive patient.

From the last part of this book, he would have learned how to make the Medical Establishment respond to his health needs as he, not they, defined them. He would have understood the necessity of taking responsibility for his own health, to get it back on track, *before* he got sick. He would have known how to avoid illness. But, best of all, he could have found the way to his optimum potential for well-being in body, mind, and spirit. He would have discovered for the first time in his life what it really means to be healthy.

Adam Americus is fictitious but the events in his life are not fiction. Every day our relatives and friends, women and men, adults and children, become unnecessary victims of disability and death from many diseases that can be prevented. Most of us fail to attain the fullness of life that is our birthright. Truly, changing this current American way of medicine is a matter of life or death.

PART ONE

The Medical Establishment

CHAPTER 1

Defining the Medical
Establishment

TODAY, the Medical Establishment is big business, a conglomerate of organized medicine, hospitals, pharmaceutical manufacturers, and health insurance companies. It is the second largest industry in the United States, generating almost 10% of the gross national product—and growing bigger each year.

The Medical Establishment provided $287 billion worth of goods and services last year, whether we needed them or not. One in seven Americans was hospitalized and, on any one day, over a million beds were occupied. In 1981, there were 36,494,000 admissions to the nation's 5,879 community hospitals for an average stay of 7.6 days at a daily cost of $332.10. Our total hospital bill was $118 billion (a 17.5% increase over 1980).

Most of us saw a physician five times during the year, for which we paid $55 billion in fees and for which our doctors gave us, among other things, prescriptions for 5 billion tranquilizers.

(Whether we write 1,000,000,000 or spell out *billion*, we usually don't stop to consider just how much that is. A trillion may cause us to pause a minute, but a billion seems to roll off our tongues with no thought. Yet consider: If you spend a dollar a *second*, it will take thirty-two years—until the year 2015—to spend a billion dollars. It has been only one billion *minutes* since the birth of Christ; and one billion *hours* ago, there was no human life on Earth.)

We rarely stop to think about the magnitude of the Medical Establishment or ask how much we know about this system in which we have placed all our faith and which we permit to make all our health decisions. To the awestruck lay observer, each medical breakthrough during the past fifty years has seemed more spectacular than the one before. Our television sets have taken us into the guarded sanctums of the Medical Establishment—the physician's examining room, the operating suite, the delivery room, even the morgue where an autopsy is taking place. We have been impressed, as well as overwhelmed, by the authority of the medical team and the knowledge it has of things we know so little about.

We've been brainwashed. We've been made to feel inadequate to judge anything medical. What we have seen from a distance has frightened us. We have been made to feel as we do when we look under the hood of a new car and realize that if something goes wrong, we won't have the vaguest notion of how to correct it. We are thankful that there are mechanics who have been trained to diagnose and fix parts that may break down. But we feel helpless.

As a result of this deep sense of inadequacy and helplessness, most of us have given up responsibility for our own health—assured that when we break down the Medical Establishment will know how to fix us. After all, there is now a specialist for every one of our parts. There is, however, a growing concern. We know the Medical Establishment is capable of providing the best medical care the world has ever seen. But the questions many of our people have begun to ask are: Will we be able to get the care we need when we need it? And if we do have access to care, will we be able to afford it?

For the estimated 50 million people with no form of health insurance, access to needed care is a pressing issue, although the problem of access is not limited to those who are financially disenfranchised. The geographic distribution of physicians limits access for those who live in rural America and in the inner cities. There are several counties in rural Mississippi, for example, where no physician practices. Most physicians live and work in the more affluent suburban areas, which are consequently oversupplied. Thus there is a scarcity of physicians where the need is greatest—those areas where poorer housing, less education, and higher unemployment increase the risk of disease.

Access to medical care is further restricted by the failure of the Medical Establishment to provide adequate primary care—the level of care that can be provided by a generalist, the family physician, and which does not require referral to a specialist. (It is estimated that 80% of episodes of illness for which patients seek the services of a physician can be classified as primary care and could best be handled by a well-trained family practitioner.)

Overspecialization has resulted in a shortage of family physicians, so that 60% of primary care today is provided by specialists who are neither trained for, nor interested in, the myriad mundane problems of this level of care.

Even the medical schools and other big city hospitals generally do a poor job of providing primary care. In most, the specialty clinic systems, manned by specialists, are called upon to provide primary care. For patients with multiple problems, this care is fragmented, slow, and costly. Patients are shunted to a different specialty clinic for each of their problems, they often have to wait weeks between appointments, and many are forced to use the expensive hospital emergency room for much of their primary medical care.

The high cost of medical care severely limits access to medical service for the poor and the elderly and is increasingly limiting access for all segments of the population, even the affluent. There are several other factors contributing to the escalating cost. These include: 1) an increased percentage of the elderly in our population who require more care than younger individuals; 2) general inflation; and 3) the ability to provide a greater depth of care as our knowledge and technology have grown. This last element has become associated with an understandable motivation on the part of physicians known as the *technological imperative*. Simply stated, most physicians believe that if it is technically possible to do something for a patient, it should be done, no matter what the cost. This has become the most important factor in cost escalation, and the most controversial, because it produces a moral dilemma for many conscientious physicians. *We have reached the point where physicians are providing more specialized and costly care than the American people need.* Much of this care involves the use of very sophisticated, high-technology equipment that requires large capital outlays and high day-to-day cost of technicians to run and maintain it.

In many instances this high-technology care has life-and-death implications for the relatively few who require it—intensive care nurseries for premature babies, renal dialysis centers, and cardiac surgery units, for example—creating a moral dilemma for those who oppose allocation of resources for it. The situation is compounded by the excess number of specialists practicing in these high-technology fields, far exceeding the needs of the American public. Some specialists are 200% in excess of the need. Many of these physicians, because there is no place for them in large medical centers, work in smaller hospitals where they become "potboiler" specialists, literally sitting around waiting for a case to come in. Often these benched specialists are forced into a form of incompetence that is the reverse of the Peter Principle: They are required to provide care which is below their level of competence and capability and for which they are not trained. For example, when a specialist is forced to provide primary care it is frequently inadequate and the patient is charged a much higher fee than a family physician would charge for the same treatment. In addition, specialists tend to order more costly laboratory tests and other ancillary services. On the other hand, many of these same specialists never have the opportunity to see the volume of cases necessary to maintain the skills they developed in their training programs. Consequently, their specialty care rarely achieves the higher quality available in those centers that do have an adequate volume of these high-technology, high-skill procedures, such as most heart operations.

Unfortunately, many physicians equate high-technology, high-cost care with high-quality care. In most instances, this is not true. Those of us who have been intimately involved with evaluating quality of care have found that high cost is often associated with poor-quality care. Also, if the quality of care administered by different providers (physicians and/or institutions) is compared by measuring the outcome (results obtained) in healing the same condition, it is obvious that the same results can have widely different costs. Eighty percent of the time, these differences are attributable to the practice style of the physician when other causes of cost variation (such as health, status, and age of the patient population) are ruled out.*

This has led to the identification of two types of care with variation in their costs but no appreciable difference in quality. The high-cost care has been termed "elaborate" and the low-cost "conservative." More and more of our present-day care can be characterized as elaborate. Much of it is associated with high-technology methodologies but in most instances does not result in higher quality care or higher quality of life for the patient.

Most physicians are honestly unaware of their role in causing the marked escalation of health care costs. They tend to blame the hospitals, the financing of medical services, the malpractice situation, and government red tape (subjects which will be discussed later). Yet the profession's behavior in permitting our present degree of overspecialization and its endorsement of the technological imperative without concern for the cost of this elaborate care has created a health care system that is out of control.

The contemporary Medical Establishment can be characterized as a space age dinosaur whose ever-increasing appetite for technology is driving us into bankruptcy. Every day it needs to have more patients, to perform more lab tests, to prescribe more drugs, to hospitalize more bodies to fill its beds, delivery rooms, and operating suites—just to pay the rent!

Yet, the public fails to see it in this light. The Establishment, and especially its professional component, is still viewed as a sacred cow. Even government, in its attempt to control runaway costs, has failed to point a finger at the medical profession and therefore has not faced this basic cause of the problem. Instead, controls have been aimed at the hospital

* Walter McClure, Personal communication.

in the form of a ceiling on capital expenditures, per diem costs, and control of utilization. The ceiling has proved ineffective because the basic causes have been overlooked. In this matter, government still reflects the public image.

Most of us would prefer not to believe that the Medical Establishment is a wasteful, self-interested dinosaur. We want to believe that its only concern is our best interests, that it is a paragon of virtue worthy of our trust. We want to believe that all physicians and medical personnel are wise, honest, selfless, dedicated individuals motivated only to do good works and serve others. We would like to think that a doctor is available whenever we need him or her, twenty-four hours a day, seven days a week, especially on Wednesday afternoons. That this doctor is willing to get out of bed in the dark of night, in any kind of weather, to make a house call, even if we live ten miles out in the country. That all we have to do is pick this doctor's name at random out of the telephone book.

We would prefer not to acknowledge—out loud, at least—that errors are made or diagnoses missed, that drugs are often prescribed unnecessarily, and that some prescribed drugs can have dangerous side effects that will adversely affect us or our offspring, even thirty years from now. We want to believe that no unnecessary procedures are ever performed and that we are never hospitalized when we could be treated equally well as out-patients (even though our health insurance won't cover the costs unless we are hospitalized). We keep telling ourselves that our physician really cares.

Many people nostalgically remember the medical care system of the early 1900s, when the major player was the physician with a little black bag and a horse and buggy. The bag was little because little was required to practice the art of medicine—a stethoscope, a scalpel, and a few basic drugs like digitalis and morphine. The chief medical facility was the doctor's office. Most people were born and died at home; only a few saw the inside of a hospital. But would we really be willing to give up the knowledge and technology of the modern Medical Establishment for only the personal services of the family doctor whom our grandparents looked upon with such confidence?

Of course not. But most of us would also agree that the pendulum has been allowed to swing too far toward the scientific and technological aspects of medicine and needs to return to the considerate and loving care that can be provided only by physicians who have concern for their fellow human beings.

Many people have discarded the belief that the Establishment is concerned with their well-being and have struck out on their own to improve their health. Forty million people went on diets last year; health food stores are opening everywhere; jogging has become a national pastime. People are searching for the answer to health and well-being and looking for leadership. They want to reclaim their own lives. The medical profession should be willing to provide the leadership necessary to restore the Medical Establishment to where it again serves the needs of the American public.

For the first seventy years of this century, the profession did build a free enterprise system of medical care that became the pride of the world. The United States was one of the few industrialized nations to resist socialized medicine because the medical profession enjoyed the support and confidence of the people. But then the profession became too involved in its love affair with technology, and it lost its head and its heart. It began to neglect the needs of the public it was designed to serve. It conquered the infectious diseases but is losing the battle with today's big killers, the chronic diseases. It has developed an almost exclusive preoccupation with the treatment of disease to the neglect of prevention, preservation, and restoration of health—at a time when we are capable of preventing 50% of all diseases and 90% of the diseases that cause 70% of all deaths and disabilities in the United States. Unless the profession wants to lose the autonomy, the esteem, and the position it holds in the minds of the people, it must redirect its course to meet their needs.

CHAPTER 2

The Making of the American Medical Establishment

AT the turn of the century, American medicine had not yet become a profession in the true sense; it had not achieved complete control of its own destiny. There was no agreed-upon body of knowledge that could be counted on to produce consistently beneficial results. Healers of many types flourished, for society had not yet granted the university-educated physician a monopoly in the healing arts.

In 1892, discouraged with the results of the kind of medicine he had seen practiced in the Civil War, Andrew Still opened his own school of osteopathic medicine in Kirksville, Missouri. Osteopathy, which emphasized the relationship between the musculoskeletal structure and organ function, was just one of the healing arts popular at the time. Chiropractors advanced the idea that disease was caused by abnormal functioning of the nervous system and could be cured simply by manipulating the spinal column. Others advocated homeopathy, the practice of using minute doses of drugs to simulate the symptoms of the disease being treated.

Patent medicines were generally more popular than remedies prescribed by physicians, probably because they contained opium and alcohol. Traveling medicine shows, advertising snake oil nostrums, became an institution in the West. "Doctors" of all descriptions could be found, and some didn't even bother to attend one of the many proprietary medical schools, known to be easy diploma mills.

In this confused milieu it's no wonder that the public lacked confidence in any system. Most people were probably unaware of the major scientific advances in the last half of the nineteenth century. Louis Pasteur's proof of the germ theory of disease in 1862 was the most significant step forward. Coupled with the discovery of anesthesia in the mid-nineteenth century, it led to a complete revolution in the practice of surgery. Thus, in 1865, Baron Joseph Lister introduced the use of antiseptics in the operating theater—a practical consequence of Pasteur's idea. Aseptic technique was then developed to prevent contamination of the surgical wound. At first, this procedure simply involved scrubbing of the hands and steam sterilization of the sheets and towels used to drape the patient. Then came the introduction of rubber gloves by William S. Halsted in 1890 and, finally, the surgical mask by Johann von Mikulicz-Radecki in 1896. Another key advance was Wilhelm Roentgen's discovery of X rays in 1898.

But perhaps most important for American medicine was the establishment of a new form of medical education at Johns Hopkins University by William Osler. In 1888, Osler became the first professor of medicine at the new Johns Hopkins School of Medicine. (Later, in 1911, he was knighted while holding the Regius Chair of Medicine at Oxford.) William S. Halsted was professor of surgery; Howard A. Kelly, chief of obstetrics and gynecology; and William H. Welsh, chief of pathology. These four men created a pattern of clinical teaching that was to become the model for all American medical schools. The curriculum was based on the study of anatomy, physiology, chemistry, bacteriology, and pathology. Use of the laboratory was encouraged and teaching was extended to patients on the wards. The first students enrolled in 1892. Years were to pass, however, before this American model was recognized.

For the first decades of the twentieth century, Germany and Austria continued to be the centers of medical education. Most American doctors-to-be wanted to take their entire medical training abroad. If this was not possible, then they tried to spend some time in postgraduate study at a European clinic, since this was viewed as almost essential for a successful career in the U.S.

Then, the Carnegie Foundation for the Advancement of Teaching established a commission to study medical education in America and appointed Abraham Flexner chairman. The Flexner Report, published in 1910, became a landmark document. Each of the 155 medical schools in the United States and Canada was rated on the quality of its instruction and facilities. The impact was momentous. Many schools closed immediately and others, those that survived, restructured their curricula.

With the Flexner Report, the scientific era in American medical education began. The training of physicians shifted from an apprenticeship in the art of medicine to a university-based educational process that infused scientific knowledge into the theory and practice of caring for the sick. The Johns Hopkins method became the model for medical education and inaugurated a new age of research by the scientific method.

The graduates of this new educational process received an M.D. degree, and the body of knowledge and system of medical practice became known as allopathic medicine to distinguish it from homeopathy, because it rejected the theory that drugs would cure by simulating the symptoms of the disease being treated. Osteopathy was frowned on (although, later, osteopathy would incorporate all the principles of allopathic medicine in its educational institutions and practice). Chiropractors were equated with quacks and were shunned; it would be unethical for a respectable M.D. to associate with a charlatan. Even the patent medicines, elixirs, and tonics began to disappear from the pharmacy shelves. Prescription drugs, written in Latin by the physician and concocted in mystery by the pharmacist, replaced the old home remedies.

American medicine had entered its new scientific era, but the vision of medicine as an art had not been lost. The family physician who retained a concerned bedside manner was accorded a place near to God in our culture. Apollo smiled on this skilled descendant of Hippocrates.

Credit must be given to the American Medical Association (AMA) for implementing the Flexner Report and bringing about this radical change in American medicine. Over the next thirty years, the medical profession moved to consolidate and secure its new status as one of the most highly regarded occupations in the land. This task was made easier by the way the profession had organized the AMA, its professional association.

No physician was permitted to have direct membership in the AMA. Membership began in a county medical society, at the community level where the physician sought to practice. Acceptance was determined by the local society, but there was a general understanding that any reputable and ethical licensed M.D. was eligible for membership. The medical school conferred the M.D. degree, the state determined licensure, but the county medical society decided who was reputable and ethical. Only recently has the AMA permitted direct membership, but the political base remains at the grass roots.

The county society selects delegates to the House of Delegates at the state level and the state society selects delegates to the House of Delegates at the national level. Delegates are selected by a nominating committee appointed by the presidents of the county and state societies. Since electioneering is forbidden, it is difficult to oppose the slate of officers and delegates selected by the nominating committee. Reelection as a delegate is common, so that new blood is infused into the leadership of the organization only very slowly.

Since the national AMA House of Delegates selects the officers and Board of Trustees—the governing and policy-making body that acts between the semiannual meetings of the House of Delegates—the AMA is a politically stable organization. Policy is difficult to challenge or change without the consent of the ruling oligarchy. (I call it an oligarchy because relatively few physicians, considering the total number of M.D.'s, are politically active in the AMA, and even fewer are in a position to exert political influence.)

This political disengagement—if not disenfranchisement—has not generally concerned most physicians. Their first concern has been their practice, which of course includes their patients. Most joined the AMA only because they felt they had to—a fact of professional life, like needing a license in order to practice. And in the early days AMA membership was a necessity; hospital privileges, the ability to get insurance, even the right to join the navy were dependent on AMA membership. Consequently, until the 1960s, nearly every practicing M.D. was a member of the AMA.

The AMA came to speak for the profession. There is no other organization; the AMA alone represents the physician. And it has become the most powerful trade association in America, more powerful than any union. The AMA *is* organized medicine. Even today, with the many medical specialty societies, there is no doubt as to whose voice speaks for the profession.

It was the AMA that secured the autonomy of the profession, its right of self-determination, its freedom from strict government control. It was the AMA's Council on Medical Education that approved the medical schools and their curricula. In later years, when the medical schools became well established and formed the Association of American Medical Colleges, a joint committee with the Council of Medical Education, called the Liaison Committee on Medical Education, was set up to assume this function. This mechanism persists today as the means of accrediting medical schools.

At the state level, the AMA, through its component state medical societies, is usually asked to nominate physicians to serve on the state licensing boards. It is this position in controlling medical licensure that has allowed the AMA to determine the standards of medical practice and to bar those it feels are not professionally qualified. One consequence is that in most states chiropractors are licensed only for those activities not likely to harm a client, in the opinion of the AMA. Restrictions have also been placed on the paramedical professionals who work with physicians in caring for patients. Under the licensing laws, these health professionals must carry out their activities "under the supervision of a licensed physician." In other words, such professionals as nurses, physical therapists, clinical psychologists, and pharmacists cannot set up a totally independent practice.

Over the years, the AMA has also been a powerful force in determining health legislation. Few health bills have been passed that the AMA has opposed, and none has cruised unnoticed on its path through the legislative process. Of all the health organizations, the AMA, through its political action committee (AMPAC), was the largest contributor to the campaign funds of political candidates in the 1980 elections.* In fact, it ranked third among all contributors; only the National Association of Realtors and the United Auto Workers put more into the politicians' coffers.

Organized medicine has clearly created a monopoly for the M.D. as the legitimate healer in American society. Legislation enacted over the years to protect the profession's position has almost assured the continuation of this enviable status. While a profession's position is always subject to the public's approval, quite apart from acceptance by the state, most people have been dazzled by the predictability and success of modern medicine. Indeed, until recently the public would have sided with the profession in any dispute the AMA might have had with the government. It is in large part for this reason that American medicine has evaded all attempts to socialize medical care, even though most industrialized countries in the world, including Canada, have nationalized their health care industries.

The AMA's concern, however, has not been solely to secure its own autonomy. Its goal has been to raise the quality of medical care in the United States, and preservation of its monopoly on healing has been seen as a means of achieving that goal. Even before the Flexner Report, the AMA was concerned with establishing minimal standards for health services. In 1906, for example, it sponsored the passage of the Pure Food and Drug Act. The Food and Drug Administration, the governmental agency that administers this law, has become responsible for maintaining high standards for drug manufacture, food processing, and the marketing of therapeutic devices.

One area where the AMA's activity has been quite limited, however, is the field of public health; that is, the organized community effort in

---

* Candidates from both parties received support if they were politically conservative (more Republicans than Democrats met this criterion). Senator John Tower (R.–Tex.) must have been seen as the most conservative; he received $20,000. Senators Howard Baker (R.–Tenn.) and Jesse Helms (R.–N.C.) both got $14,000. Robert Dole (R.–Kan.), the chairman of the Senate Finance Committee—which acts on most health legislation—received $12,000, and his counterpart in the House, Dan Rostenkowski (D.–Ill.), chairman of the Ways and Means Committee, got $9,500.

the promotion of health and the prevention of disease. The AMA would like to remain the ultimate *authority* in the whole field of health but limit its *activity* to the practice of medicine. It sees the provision of public health services as a responsibility of governmental agencies at the local, state, and national levels.

This, of course, has created confusion in the meaning of *health care* and *medical care*, terms many use interchangeably. Medical care is perhaps best defined as the professional care provided by a physician. In practice, medical care is often confined to the diagnosis and treatment of disease, but it should include the preservation and restoration of health as well as the prevention of disease. Although many physicians do incorporate the prevention of disease into their practice, most ignore their responsibility for the preservation and restoration of health. I would define health as a state of complete physical, mental, emotional, and social well-being. Most physicians, however, define health as the absence of disease, making it something beyond their interest, training, and area of expertise.

Health care is a term that is commonly misused. In the strict sense, it should apply only to those services designed to preserve and restore a state of complete physical, mental, emotional, and social well-being. In vernacular usage, however, it refers to any healing service provided by a nonphysician, to differentiate it from services provided by physicians (medical care). A hospital, for example, is a health care institution. As a corporate entity separate from its medical staff, it cannot be licensed to practice medicine (the diagnosis and treatment of disease) but it does provide care for the sick, hence "health care."

It is easy to understand why physicians have come to give almost exclusive attention to the diagnosis and treatment of disease at the expense of concern with the health of their patients. For, like the public in general, physicians have been enthralled by the rapidly expanding knowledge of disease. The new science-oriented physician has so much to learn that attention to anything other than the diagnosis and treatment of disease may seem a neglect of his or her professional responsibility. The AMA, with its insistence on the autonomy and authority of the profession, has tended to foster this split between medical and health care.

The AMA has had a vital interest in the socioeconomics of medical care and especially the organization of medical practice. It's "Principles of Medical Ethics" was based on a system of fee-for-service solo practice, a model that was almost universal in the first few decades of the twentieth century. Thus, in those early years, organized medicine could concentrate on establishing control of the system of medical education and the education of paramedical professionals, the licensing of all health workers, and developing a powerful lobby in health legislation.

Having established minimal standards of education and licensure, the AMA relied on its constituent societies at the county medical society level to voluntarily control the quality of medical care. The individual physician, having met the profession's minimum standards, was free to practice according to his own conscience under the watchful eye of his peers.

CHAPTER 3

Surgeons:
A Breed Apart

THE AMERICAN MEDICAL ASSOCIATION did much to secure the autonomy of the profession and its responsibility for its own regulation. But it was not the only organization involved. Within the medical world, surgeons as a group have been instrumental in establishing guidelines for the proper practice of their art.

Even at the time of the Flexner Report, surgery was emerging as a distinct specialty, a practice apart from general medicine. In 1910, a congress of surgeons was held in Chicago. Three years later, in 1913, these men founded the American College of Surgeons, whose objective, as stated in its Articles of Incorporation, was: "To maintain an association of surgeons, not for pecuniary profit, but for the benefit of humanity by advancing the science of surgery and the ethical and competent practice of its art."

But in the early days of this specialty, the science and the art were still primitive. The surgeon was not free to perform many procedures he knew he would be technically capable of. Other factors interfered. The persistent barrier was shock; surgeons were limited by the trauma of the surgery itself, by the stress that the body could withstand. Despite antiseptic and aseptic techniques, infection was a constant threat. Anesthesia was still imperfect, and the danger mounted with every minute the patient was anesthetized. The deeper the anesthesia, the more relaxed the muscles, permitting better access to the depths of the abdominal cavity but also bringing the patient closer to death.

◄§ It is 1915. Eager medical students crowd the tiers of wooden benches that rise steeply in concentric circles above the operating theater. A hushed, rustling sound is heard as they shift their feet nervously and converse in hoarse whispers. Dawn is breaking and the frost on the panes of the skylight takes on a pink hue.

A nurse in a long blue skirt and a starched white apron backs in through the left side of the double swinging doors. Instantly the theater is quiet. She opens the door of one of the two glass-and-enamel instrument cabinets that stand side by side against the six-foot-high wall that completely rings the theater.

Twenty-one pairs of eyes follow her every move. She picks out several ivory-handled scalpels, some forged steel scissors, and a large number of Kelly hemostats (a clamplike instrument used to stop bleeding) and places them on her tray. The steel on steel makes a hollow clang which reverberates through the amphitheater. Glancing up at the staring eyes, the nurse quickly backs out through the padded-leather swinging door on the right.

The rustling is just resuming when both doors open and a stretcher is rolled in by two orderlies and the nurse. The patient, a woman, appears obese as she lies on the stretcher, covered, except for her head, with a white cotton blanket. Her face is scarlet. The nurse helps her slide onto the wooden operating table, which has been draped with a white sheet, while the orderlies keep the stretcher from rolling away. The patient groans and begins to shake violently.

"A chill," one student says out loud, without realizing it.

"Correct," resounds a booming voice from the doorway. A tall, thin man strides into the theater. He is dressed in a white gown that falls to his knees, with his striped morning pants, gray spats, and black shoes protruding below. The wooden floor creaks as he circles the operating table, drying his hands with a towel. His full beard is only partially concealed by the gauze mask that covers his mouth and chin. His pince-nez balances on the bridge of his nose. Gazing over the top of his glasses, he addresses the rows of students.

"Our patient this morning is indeed having a chill. She is forty-one years of age, the mother of five, and you will notice she is somewhat overweight. She was admitted to the hospital last night with severe pain in her abdomen that radiated to her back on the right side. Oh yes, she had just finished a large supper of corned beef and cabbage."

Another nurse, gowned, gloved, and masked, holds a rubber glove open by its inverted cuff. The surgeon deftly slips his hand into the glove as she turns the cuff up over his gowned forearm. The other hand is similarly gloved, and he works his fingers into the tips as he continues to speak.

"It was obvious to me that she was suffering acute biliary colic, which of course suggests a gallstone problem. She presented the classic description of one predisposed to this disease: fair, fat, and forty. I could feel a tender mass in the right upper quadrant, although she had involuntary guarding of her abdominal wall which made palpation [diagnosis by touch] difficult.

"You may start the anesthetic, Miss Jackson," the surgeon now instructs a third nurse, who then proceeds to drip a liquid into the gauze-covered strainer she holds over the patient's nose and mouth. She speaks to the woman in low tones the students cannot hear. The odor of chloroform permeates the room.

"I ordered a roentgenogram, an X-ray plate, of the abdomen, which revealed an opaque shadow the size and shape of a bird's egg. I have no doubt that this is a gallstone that is impacted in the neck of the gallbladder, and it is responsible for her acute symptoms.

"It is important in these cases to operate as quickly as possible, before infection sets in and pus accumulates—in other words, before she develops an empyema. If that happens, you cannot safely remove the gallbladder and you are forced to simply drain it. A cholecystectomy, removing the gallbladder, is much cleaner. Her beginning chill indicates that we are operating none too soon."

The surgeon begins to paint the abdomen with tincture of iodine. He then soaks towels and sheets in a carbolic solution and covers all the skin except for a two-inch-wide strip down the middle. The familiar odor of the antiseptic wafts up into the gallery.

"Scalpel!" He cuts through the entire abdominal wall with one stroke. More carbolic-soaked towels are placed over the wound edges. They turn red. Large curved retractors are inserted into the abdominal cavity so that the wound can be held open by an assistant.

"Kelly!" The instrument nurse slaps the hemostat into his outstretched palm and he immediately clamps it onto the fundus of the gallbladder.

"Scissors!" Again the slapping sound. Two cuts are made on either side of the gallbladder, and then, with his index finger, he strips it from its bed on the undersurface of the liver.

"Kelly!" He peers into the depths of the wound. His pince-nez slips from his nose and follows his gaze.

"Kelly!" He reaches into the wound and retrieves his glasses, placing them again on his nose.

"Scissors!" A quick snip and the gallbladder is held up for the class to see. It has been only seven minutes since he made the incision.

"Speed and dexterity," he explains to the students, with no mention of the pince-nez, "are necessary attributes of the surgeon. It is the only way to prevent shock. We will pack the liver bed with iodoform gauze, place a drain, and get out."

The surgeon strips off his gloves as another assistant takes his place at the table and begins to suture the wound. He then takes the gallbladder, with the Kelly hemostat still attached, places it in a pan and cuts into its wall. Green bile spreads over the white enamel pan and the plink of a stone on the pan can be heard. He lifts the stone out of the bile and holds it up between his thumb and index finger for all to see as he strides around the ring of the amphitheater like a matador displaying an ear he has been awarded.

"The size of a robin's egg; the roentgenogram was right. Gentlemen, another life has been saved by the miracle of modern surgery."

He bows to the class, turns, and walks swiftly out of the room.

The gallery breaks into applause. ॐ

Only with the experience of World War I did surgeons learn how to overcome those tenacious obstructors of definitive surgery: infection and shock. Surgery on the battlefield was a world apart from the relative cleanliness of even the primitive operating theater of the early twentieth century. All wounds were contaminated, and deaths from infection, especially gas gangrene and tetanus (lockjaw), were rampant in the first year of the war. Through the sheer number of cases, however, doctors quickly learned that if, soon after the injury, the wound was adequately debrided —if all dead tissue was removed by surgical means—then infection was much less likely. The newly available tetanus antitoxin also worked much better in cases that were debrided well.

The war highlighted the need to deal with shock and thus, ironically, stimulated research in this area. Shock, it was discovered, involves a temporary loss of effective circulating blood volume and can be reversed if treated early enough; it can be prevented by the infusion of blood and other fluids. The understanding of fluid and electrolyte balance (the equilibrium of chemicals dissolved in the blood and other body fluids) was a significant breakthrough.

New and better anesthetics were developed, allowing anesthesia of longer duration and greater depth, with a wider margin of safety. This advance changed the character of surgical technique. Speed was no longer essential. Tissues could be handled more gently, blood loss could be meticulously controlled, and more complete anatomical dissection of tissues became possible, even in the depths of the abdomen. Moreover, with this new technique, the likelihood of shock was reduced and wounds healed better, with less risk of infection.

Surgery established itself as a crucial lifesaving art in the eyes of the public. And it became a far more profitable form of practice than general medicine. Unfortunately, this gain in stature was used to advantage by some unscrupulous physicians, to the detriment of the patient. Unjustified operations were performed and exorbitant fees charged. Ghost surgery was conducted by someone unknown to the patient, without the patient's consent. Fee splitting brought kickbacks and other inducements to family physicians to refer patients to a specific surgeon. In some cases, itinerant surgeons operated and then left the postoperative care of the patient to the family doctor.

The local county medical societies seemed incapable of eliminating these unethical practices, but the American College of Surgeons, through its Board of Regents, took a firm and vigilant stand against such practices. Its power was limited, however. It could discipline only its own members or deny fellowship to unethical surgeons. Consequently, its control was incomplete; in fact, many of these outlawed practices have continued to exist, although to a much limited extent. Francis D. Moore of Boston, first vice-president of the college, responding publicly to the press in 1970 when the profession was charged with permitting unnecessary surgery, had to explain that nearly half the surgery in the U.S. was still being performed by physicians who were not board-certified surgeons or fellows of the college.

Despite its lack of complete control, the American College of Surgeons has had a positive impact on the quality of surgical care. Fellowship in the college carries prestige not only in America but throughout the world. The letters F.A.C.S. after a physician's name provide a certain guarantee. Only physicians who limit their practice to a surgical specialty and who have had approved surgical training and education can become fellows of the college. They must possess ethical standards and their professional competence must be attested to by fellows who are familiar with their work. All fellows sign a pledge to practice their profession with dedication, placing the well-being of their patients above all else and serving all people with skill and fidelity. Every fellow is subject to discipline by the college.

One way the American College of Surgeons extended its control over the practice of surgery was by establishing a hospital standardization program in 1918. Since surgeons require the facilities and services of a hospital to practice their profession, they need to be sure that the hospital they use will provide for optimal patient care. They need to know, for instance, that instruments will be adequately sterilized, that the operating suite does not harbor bacteria, that the results of laboratory tests will be accurate, and that their patients will receive good nursing care at all times. In the early days, these conditions varied from hospital to hospital. Thus, the college sought to establish minimum standards that could be relied on by its members.

This method of quality control was based on the assumption that if the environment in which care was provided was good—for example, if a particular hospital met all the standards—then the care provided by that hospital would be good. This simple and naive approach worked and the quality of care improved. (It was not until the 1970s that measurements of performance as well as standards for the environment were incorporated into quality control measurements; they revealed that a good environment per se did not assume high quality, a subject to be discussed later.)

The improvement in hospital conditions marked the beginning of a trend that was to assign key importance to the hospital in the health care system. By the 1970s, the hospital had become the coordinating center of a community's health care, usually the only place in the community where medical services could be obtained on an emergency basis, twenty-four hours a day, seven days a week.

But in the early 1920s, only surgeons relied on the hospital for their livelihood. Indeed, it was the surgeon who was responsible for the establishment of the emergency room or accident ward, as it was usually called, because it was meant to handle traumatic injuries rather than the general medical conditions that were to be treated in the physicians' offices.

In 1922, the American College of Surgeons' Committee on Trauma was organized to develop programs to improve the care of the injured. And until the recent development of the specialty of emergency medicine, it was the surgical service of a hospital that was responsible for staffing the emergency room.

As medical knowledge and technology grew, the little black bag had to expand to include an ever-increasing armamentarium. It became easier to bring the patient to the little black bag than vice versa. "Meet me at the accident ward" became the physician's instruction to a patient in an emergency.

More and more specialists found that the cost of new equipment was too much for an individual physician to afford. To avoid duplication of expensive instruments and machines, they followed the surgeons' lead and asked the hospital to become the community resource, providing staff members with the latest technological innovations. The hospitals were only too glad to fulfill this role because they wanted to attract physicians' practices to their institutions. Soon, internists and other medical specialists were copying surgeons with their hospital-centered form of practice.

By 1952, the American College of Surgeons had been joined by the American College of Physicians, the American Medical Association, and the American Hospital Association in its hospital standardization program. Together, these groups formed a new organization, the Joint Commission on Accreditation of Hospitals (JCAH), to develop and monitor the quality standards of the nation's health care institutions. The JCAH, as an instrument of the private sector, was a uniquely American institution; it was a voluntary effort by the various interests of the profession to provide a formal mechanism to regulate the nation's hospitals. Its success, and that of the American College of Surgeons' program before it, must be credited with keeping government control at a minimum in the health field. With the freedom of self-regulation, which of course must go hand in hand with responsibility, the profession built a system of hospital care for America that was to be the best the world had ever seen.

CHAPTER 4

Hospitals and Health Insurance
Color the Picture

MOST HOSPITALS in America are community hospitals. They are also referred to in the trade as short-term general hospitals, since the average length of stay is about a week and they handle all kinds of illness and injury. The 1982 *Guide to the Health Care Field*, published by the American Hospital Association, lists 5,879 such hospitals. Of these, 1,794 are owned and operated by local or state governments, and 729 are investor-owned for-profit hospitals. The large majority (3,356), however, are nonprofit community hospitals, most of which (about 2,500) were built before World War II.

Although some nonprofit community hospitals are owned and operated by religious organizations—the largest number by the Catholic Church—most were organized by a local group of interested citizens who obtained a charter from the state giving them the authority to operate a hospital. The trustees of these hospitals are usually laypeople, unschooled in health matters but concerned that their community have the finest in medical and health care.

This lay board of trustees relies on a medical staff to provide medical care and on an administrative staff to manage nursing care and other necessary support services. In the United States, the board itself usually hires the key administrators and thus controls the administration of the hospital. But it has had to work out a more tenuous arrangement with the medical profession, which insists on its autonomy even within the hospital.

Many of the existing arrangements, whether formal or informal, would be impossible to diagram on the usual organizational chart. The late Ray Brown, one of America's most knowledgeable hospital administrators, likened the typical hospital organization to a three-legged organism (board, administration, and medical staff) without a head. This arrangement, he said, often resulted in a three-way standoff, with each leg trying to carry the organization in its own direction. Usually, he had to admit, the medical staff won.

The typical board member is a local philanthropist or a representative of the "old money" in the community that paid for the first building, endowed the new operating room, or continually headed the list of contributors to the annual fundraising drive. Most boards are self-perpetuating, and their members serve for life. Even though philanthropy currently provides less than 6% of the hospital's support, the board composition remains the same.

In the early days, the board usually employed a physician or a nurse as superintendent of the hospital. But this professional often had no training in finance, business, or management. In time, other arrangements had to be made. Some boards chose one of their own to be the "managing director" of the hospital; frequently this was a board member who had retired from the family business and needed something to do. Thus, the hospital came to be run like the family firm. Although today such a situation might seem ludicrous, it was a common setup until after World War II, when a cadre of trained hospital administrators became available.

Managing a hospital is totally different from running a commercial business, where the objective is control to ensure uniform quality in a specific product. In a hospital there is no one product, and each patient requires individual treatment. Management must encourage individual initiative and provide the environment necessary to facilitate and support this kind of service. The skilled administrator has to perform a careful juggling act, providing the kind of environment that facilitates individualized service with one hand while meeting operational costs and upholding general standards of care with the other.

All this was more easily accomplished in the early days. Then, hospitals had charitable immunity from prosecution for negligence; only physicians could be held responsible for the care they provided. Physicians thus made sure that the hospitals conformed to their standards (the American College of Surgeons' hospital standardization program was one result of this situation). In essence, the hospital began as the physician's workshop. It grew only as the tools physicians needed to ply their trade became more and more complex.

In the first three decades of the twentieth century, hospitals rose willy-nilly on the American landscape. There was no plan. As a community grew, it wanted its own physicians and its physicians wanted their own hospital. Community pride was an important factor, and "keeping up with the Joneses" created a uniformity in hospitals throughout the country. The latest equipment was placed in every hospital, regardless of its size. During the 1920s, cost was no concern; every medium-sized community had its own fully equipped hospital by the time Wall Street crashed in 1929.

The Great Depression brought a halt to hospital expansion, but it gave birth to a third component of the Medical Establishment—the health insurance industry. Until this time, medical and hospital bills alike were paid out of the patient's pocket on a fee-for-service basis. There was no health insurance as we know it today. As the Depression deepened, however, hospitals found that most of their patients could not pay for the care they needed.

In 1932, the American Hospital Association organized a nonprofit prepayment plan called Blue Cross, in order to assure its members that they would at least recover the cost of services provided. This plan was modeled after one that had been operating since 1929 in Dallas, Texas. By paying a monthly fee in advance, a group of schoolteachers had contracted with Baylor University Hospital to provide hospital care should they need it. The fee was paid whether or not the individual teacher ever used the services. By spreading the risk over a number of schoolteachers, the hospital could afford to provide care if and when it was needed.

Thus, prepaid health insurance was born, with a fiscal intermediary between the subscriber to the plan and the hospital. The intermediary collected an actuarially determined fixed fee from the subscriber to cover specific benefits, and it reimbursed the hospital on the basis of its costs. The intermediary had no role in controlling costs; if costs increased, the intermediary simply passed these on to the subscriber in the form of increased premiums the following year.

Cost reimbursement was instituted innocently during those Depression years. The not-for-profit hospitals were considered charitable institutions, interested only in recovering their costs. Over the years, however, this reimbursement mechanism has served as a blank check to the hospital industry, and it has been the principal cause of inflation in the cost of hospital care. Hospitals have been able to increase the number of employees, raise wages, add more beds, and purchase expensive new equipment—knowing that these outlays would be reimbursed. This rise in the supply side of the economic equation has pushed up costs. And in the economics of health care, if the supply side increases, demand will soon follow. If it is there, it will be used.

Because the cost reimbursement system of financing required no change in the organization of the health care delivery system, organized medicine readily embraced the concept. In fact, it developed a similar plan of its own to cover physicians' fees—the prepayment plan known as Blue Shield. Blue Shield plans were usually organized by state medical societies. Although Blue Cross and Blue Shield were separate entities, they were frequently marketed to the public as a combined Blue Cross/Blue Shield package of health insurance.

Blue Shield required a fee schedule, something that organized medicine had always opposed. But this appeared to be the lesser of two evils. Voluntary health insurance was seen by the AMA as a possible deterrent to the national health insurance plan that was being advocated as part of the New Deal, the same program that instituted Social Security. It also pushed back the specter of socialized medicine, which was looming in Europe.

The Blue Shield fee schedule was developed on the basis of usual, customary, and reasonable charges. *Usual* referred to an individual physician's fees, based on his or her training, experience, and skills. A particular bill was to reflect what the physician usually charged for that procedure, with everyone in the same economic level being charged the same fee. *Customary* referred to the amount that it was customary to charge in a specific geographic location by physicians with similar training, experience, and skills. *Reasonable* referred to a fee for an unusual case, one with complications or special problems that required the expenditure of more than the usual time. In these cases, any increased fee was to be commensurate with the degree of difficulty.

This fee schedule has worked to the advantage of physicians and the public alike. Over the years it has kept fees in line and prevented the escalation in costs seen in hospitals. For the physician, it has meant that fee-for-service individual practice could continue.

Commercial insurance companies soon followed the lead of the "Blues" and developed policies to cover medical care. Like Blue Cross, which had been designed to insure (or, more correctly, to prepay) hospital care alone, these commercial plans at first covered only in-hospital services, excluding ambulatory and preventive care. The commercial companies did not believe it would be actuarially sound to insure care provided in a physician's office, as proper monitoring of the use of insurance benefits seemed possible only when the care was given in a hospital. What this stipulation led to, however, was an increase in unnecessary hospitalization. Many physicians found it difficult to resist the cry of patients who insisted on being hospitalized just so their insurance would cover the cost of treatment.

Unlike the Blues, however, commercial health insurance was not a prepayment plan. It dealt directly with patients, indemnifying them for the risk of having to pay for medical care. It was a true insurance program, based on actuarial risk. Unlike Blue Cross/Blue Shield, payment was made to the patient, not to the hospital or the doctor. Reimbursement for hospital care was a set amount, based on hospital charges, not costs. The basis for reimbursement varied with different policies and for different insurance companies. Reimbursement might be based on a specific amount for the care of a specific disease or for the performance of a specific procedure, but more often it was based on a specific amount per day, irrespective of the services provided. The patient was reimbursed in the same manner for the care provided by a physician.

Because indemnity coverage by commercial insurance companies, unlike Blue Cross, did not vary with the amount of care or the number of services provided, it did not tend to cause the same inflationary increase in the cost of hospital care. But in order to compete with Blue Cross, the commercial companies had to raise their prices as hospital costs increased over the years.

Both the Blue Cross/Blue Shield and commercial health insurance companies have become third parties in the health marketplace, positioned between the patient and the providers of health care services. Because the third parties pay for the care the patient receives, many believe the patient no longer acts as a prudent buyer. With little concern for the price charged by various providers (*i.e.*, "My insurance will cover it"), there is no incentive to find care at a cheaper rate, thereby removing competition and the effect it has on controlling costs. There is no competition; therefore, there is no marketplace economy in health care. It would be different, some say, if people had to pay out of their pockets. But few would be willing now to give up health insurance.

Another system of financing also began during the Depression—the consumer cooperative movement. In rural America, in particular, groups of consumers organized plans that hired physicians to provide medical care services on a fixed salary. These cooperatives charged their members a predetermined fixed fee. Similar schemes were initiated by groups of physicians. The Ross-Loos Clinic in Los Angeles was probably the first prepaid group practice plan.

Industry, too, began to set up prepaid medical care plans. Kaiser Industries asked Dr. Sidney Garfield to form a group practice to provide medical services for workers building the Grand Coulee Dam in the state of Washington. During World War II, similar arrangements were made to provide medical services for Kaiser employees at various new war plants located at a distance from established sources of health care (see Chapter 10).

Organized medicine fought this encroachment on fee-for-service individual practice from the start. The first prepaid group practice plans were vigorously attacked as a communist-inspired invasion of the practice of medicine. Physicians who joined such groups were expelled from county and state medical societies and from the AMA. Industry-based groups were derided for offering "contract medicine," and it was considered un-ethical for a physician to work "for hire" in such groups.

Since states, not the federal government, have jurisdiction over the practice of medicine, the AMA lobbied to have state legislatures enact laws forbidding the corporate practice of medicine. *Corporate practice* referred to any arrangement by which an organization collected the fees for a physician's services and in turn paid the physician a salary. (The term applied only to direct patient care by the physician. A physician was permitted to work in an administrative capacity for an organization since the organization would not be collecting fees for the physician's patient-care services.) Twenty-two states eventually passed such restrictive legis-lation, which further helped to entrench fee-for-service, solo practice of medicine.

Whatever the reimbursement plan, by the beginning of Word War II, the importance of the hospital in American medicine was well established. The medical profession had brought a large percentage of its practice into the hospital. Although nearly all primary care was still centered in the family doctor's office, secondary care by specialists was well under way, often requiring the use of sophisticated equipment in the hospital. The medical school hospitals were beginning to be recognized as tertiary care institutions, with superspecialists providing treatment that could not be given in a community hospital. Yet, still ruling the roost, the kings in the local hospital, were the great general surgeons.

~§ It is 1940 and this is John Cleaver's fourth year as a medical stu-dent. He is on his surgical clerkship in a suburban community hospital that has a loose affiliation with his medical school. He has been on the surgical service for two weeks and has grown accustomed to being scrubbed all morning. On this particular day, the chief is helping the resident-in-training take out a gallbladder.

John glances at the wall clock. An hour on this case, he notes. His hands feel permanently bent to the shape of the handles of the Deaver retractors he is holding. He looks about the stark, white-tiled operating room. It is beginning to get hot under the large light that is focused into the depths of the wound. His eyes catch those of the pretty student nurse who is circulating. He can tell she is smiling at him behind her mask, and he winks. She comes over and sponges the beads of perspira-tion from his brow.

"That's right, Miss Johnson, Mr. Cleaver is the only one doing manual labor this morning. Cleaver, if our anesthesiologist would relax the patient a little more, you wouldn't have to pull so hard."

The anesthesiologist stands up and peers over the screen to check the degree of relaxation. He studies his machine and examines the patient's reflexes.

"Mr. Cleaver, have I ever told you my definition of a surgeon?" asks the anesthesiologist.

"No, sir, I don't believe you have."

"Well, let me educate you. A surgeon has the courage of a lion, the hands of a woman, the eye of an eagle, and the brains of a flea." He sits down.

"I guess that means we're not going to get any more relaxation," remarks the surgeon. "Cleaver, you'll just have to keep pulling on those retractors. This is Dr. Roberts's first gallbladder, you know, and he is doing a damn good job, despite the anesthesia."

The resident's ears turn red, but he gives his chief a look of gratitude. Not knowing what to say, he asks a question: "How do I know for sure that there are no other stones, besides the one I found in the common duct?"

"You don't, for sure. But we found only one stone, the size of a pea, and that would indicate it has been there for some time. If there were others, they would have rubbed against one another, causing a wearing down of one or more sides and leaving the smooth surface we call facets. Since this one has no facets, we can assume it is a solitary stone." He looks to see if Cleaver is listening. "Do you agree, Mr. Cleaver?"

"Oh, yes, sir. But . . . well . . . at the university they would probably do an operative cholangiogram."

"Glad you brought that up. X-ray visualization of the gallbladder and bile ducts during the operation is still experimental. I can see where in some situations it would be very helpful. In fact, we are making arrangements to build an X-ray machine into our new operating suite.

"But, on the other hand, there is no real indication in this case. You have to learn to rely on your clinical judgment. We've explored the common duct, palpated it from the duodenum to the liver. As I've explained, it's a solitary unfaceted stone. And we've passed a probe larger than the stone's diameter into the duodenum.

"A cholangiogram would increase the length of our procedure. Even though our anesthesia is excellent, we don't necessarily want to prolong it. Time does increase the risk of complications, especially wound infections. And it would increase the cost to the patient. Anesthesiologists charge by the minute; did you know that, Mr. Cleaver?"

"Oh, no, sir."

"Dr. Roberts, that was a beautiful exposure of the right hepatic artery. Mr. Cleaver, remember how important it is to see everything you are doing. If Dr. Roberts hadn't exposed the right hepatic artery looping up over the cystic duct, he might have accidentally ligated it and shut off the blood supply to the right lobe of the liver.

"Dr. Roberts, did I ever tell you about the first cholecystectomy I ever saw? Well, the surgeon was a professor who prided himself on his speed. He was a flamboyant showman, but rough. His pince-nez fell into the wound, but that didn't ruffle him. He had the gallbladder out in seven minutes. But he had clamped the right hepatic artery and tented the common bile duct between two Kellys while he was removing the gallbladder. The patient died of liver failure and septicemia a week later. 'Acute yellow atrophy' they called it in those days. It wouldn't happen today." ❧

Medical science was advancing rapidly. As knowledge and technology increased, so did the need for specialization. Individual physicians could no longer practice independently; they needed to call on others to help in the care of a patient.

Word War II taught the American physician teamwork and gave birth to chemotherapy. The fourth element of the Medical Establishment, the pharmaceutical industry, came into being, poised to launch the antibiotic era.

The end of the war also marked the beginning of the golden age of American medicine.

CHAPTER 5

The Start of a
Golden Age

A GOLDEN AGE is a time of challenge, creativity, and success. It comes at a time of renewal, when what is dead has been buried and there is a rebirth of hope.

World War II rescued the American people from the Great Depression, both financially and emotionally. At the end of the war, the United States, hardly touched by the devastation, stood as the most powerful nation in the world. Whether we liked it or not, we were forced from a position of isolationism into world leadership.

Improved communication, brought about by the war, became a catalyst for the expansion of knowledge. Scientists began to form organizations, to congregate, to meet face to face, as air travel made the world smaller. The printed word was more quickly disseminated. The telephone made instant contact possible. It was as though previously we had all been individual ants, moving aimlessly without direction, and then suddenly we came together as a colony—as a scientific community with common goals. And one of the first goals was to conquer infectious diseases.

Historically, Germany was far ahead of the rest of the world in the use of chemicals to treat disease. Paul Ehrlich, a German bacteriologist, was considered the father of modern chemotherapy, the term used broadly for all drug treatments. Early in the century, he had discovered that specific body tissues have a selective affinity for certain chemicals. His discovery of arsphenamine, a synthetic arsenic compound that kills the spirochete of spyhilis, launched the German pharmaceutical industry.

The Germans had also discovered the first sulfa drug in the 1930s; they found that the red dye Prontosil was effective against streptococci. At the beginning of World War II, it was even feared that Hitler might use germ warfare because the Germans were so advanced in chemotherapy.

Then the British produced penicillin. As early as 1928, Alexander Fleming had made the serendipitous observation that penicillin mold killed his cultures of staphylococci. But it wasn't until 1938 that penicillin was shown to be a safe and effective antibacterial agent, capable of being produced commercially. The war effort gave priority to its production so that the Allied forces could have it to use. The pharmaceutical industry also began to make tetanus toxoid, the vaccine against lockjaw, in large enough quantities to immunize all Allied troops and eliminate this scourge of previous wars.

One of the most exciting advances was the discovery of streptomycin, an antibiotic that killed the bacillus of tuberculosis, in 1944. Soon after this discovery, however, the bacillus seemed to develop a resistance to streptomycin. Other bacteria began to develop a resistance to penicillin. Over the next ten years, the pharmaceutical industry devoted most of its resources to the development of new antibiotics, ones that would be effective against penicillin-resistant and streptomycin-resistant microorganisms, as well as ones of a wider spectrum that would work against other organisms that caused infectious diseases.

There appeared to be no limit to the number of "miracle drugs" the industry could discover, and bacterial infections were brought under control. Viruses, however, were another matter. They were resistant to all the antibiotics. But an answer was found in immunization.

Edward Jenner's smallpox vaccination had been effective in preventing that viral infection for a hundred years before any virus was known to exist. Research led to the development of effective vaccines against influenza, yellow fever, poliomyelitis, measles, and rubella. The 1918 influenza pandemic, which killed more than 20 million people, can never occur again because the drug industry has been able to develop a new vaccine for any new virus that may come along in time to prevent such a large-scale catastrophe.

Research in immunology, however, has not been confined to the search for ways to control viral infections. Immunization is seen as the ultimate means of preventing all infectious diseases, bacterial as well as viral. Chemotherapy, in reality, is only a stopgap method of controlling infections; the ultimate goal is to prevent all infectious diseases and thus eliminate them from the face of the earth. In 1980, for instance, the World Health Organization announced that there is no more smallpox anywhere in the world. Vaccination against smallpox is no longer necessary.

By the end of World War II, then, the four elements of the Medical Establishment were in place—the medical profession, the hospitals, the health insurance industry, and the pharmaceutical manufacturers. It was in the climate of the Cold War that these four elements took shape, forming the Medical Establishment.

The Cold War stimulated an unprecedented interest in scientific research and the development of its technology. Medicine benefited indirectly from the competition fostered by the launching of Sputnik I on October 4, 1957. The U.S. quickly gave priority to research in the hard sciences, and many discoveries had useful medical applications. Miniaturization of solid-state electronic circuits, computer technology, new inert plastics, and a myriad of other developments resulted in artificial kidneys, electronic pacemakers for the heart that could be implanted in the body, improved monitoring equipment, blood vessel replacements, and eventually organ transplants.

Automation was also applied to more mundane medical processes; for instance, the old mercury thermometers were replaced by thermocouples with electronic readouts. New gadgets and new techniques caught the imagination of professionals and administrative personnel alike. Medicine began a love affair with technology.

As the in-depth knowledge of specific areas of medicine increased, individual physicians felt compelled to limit their practice to a particular area. There was just too much to learn. It became impossible to be adequately trained in all areas of medical practice. Specialization became a necessity.

With the knowledge explosion, most physicians thought they were witnessing the death of general practice. Older physicians counseled their younger colleagues to go into a specialty. It seemed no one considered the possibility of a specialist in breadth but not in depth. And no one seemed concerned with how the profession would meet the need for primary care. The effect was devastating.

In 1945, half of all practicing physicians were in general practice, and even the 50% who had specialized were not overspecialized. Most surgeons were general surgeons; many still performed all types of operations. Most internists provided some primary care; they had not yet subspecialized. By 1970, however, only 17% of practicing physicians were in general practice. Most internists had limited their practice to adults with diseases of a particular organ system; very few provided primary care.

During the Cold War, specialization grew like a cancer rather than in an orderly manner. It grew out of proportion to the need. Everyone wanted to be a specialist. The result was serious overspecialization of the entire profession.

Many factors seemed to encourage overspecialization. The most important was the American system of medical education, specifically the method of financing medical education at the time. During the war, the government had financed medical education. Students were taken into the armed forces and the government paid their tuition. By the end of the war, the cost of a medical education was well beyond the means of most individuals. Even state governments were having difficulty in subsidizing their medical schools.

The Cold War provided the answer. Medical schools found they could meet their financial needs if they met the government's need for basic research. The mechanism for this financing was the research grant, provided by the National Institutes of Health (NIH). The money from several large NIH grants could spill over into many needed services in a medical school.

Grants, however, were not distributed according to the needs of the schools. The need of the government took priority, and the schools had to vie for the individual grants. Since grants went to the researchers who could best please and meet the needs of NIH, these individuals became important resources for a medical school. Grantsmanship became a specialty in and of itself; successful grant-getters could write their own tickets. They became the heads of departments and the full professors.

Consequently, during the golden age of medicine, medical education was in the hands of the academician-researcher. The clinician, the professor who was patient-oriented and taught the art of medicine, held a subservient position. And often clinical professors in medical schools—perhaps to refurbish their own egos—cast the local medical doctor in the role of bumbling incompetent.

In reviewing the history of a patient's illness, as documented in the medical record, instructors always seemed to blame any mistake in diagnosis or any improper treatment on the family doctor. To the impressionable medical student, the local medical doctor became the low man on the medical totem pole. Basking in the sunlight at the top was the chair of the department, the full professor. No matter how motivated students were to become general practitioners on entering medical school, they usually graduated with the belief that they *must* become specialists. There was no devious plan by medical schools to stop educating general practitioners, but the result was the same. No family doctors came off the assembly line.

The specialists themselves fueled the trend to specialization. They organized. At first, they simply formed sections within the American Medical Association. But later, they created associations of their own. These associations organized conventions and meetings to discuss the particular specialists' mutual concerns. They looked at the graduate education programs in the specialty, the site of these programs, and the body of knowledge taught. They examined the certification of candidates for the practice of the specialty and talked about surveillance of the practice.

Their concern was well intentioned. The purpose was to assure quality care in the specialty. Mechanisms were set up to accomplish this goal, and they did. But they also established each specialty as an autonomous oligarchy answerable to no one, except in acquiring the initial right to exist as a separate specialty from the AMA's Council on Medical Education.

In the United States, graduate medical education in the specialties is currently carried out in residency programs in the nation's hospitals. They are so named because the physician-in-training resides in the hospital where he or she is receiving this education. Hospitals are selected for these residency programs by a residency review committee of the specialty. Graduates are certified for practice of the specialty by specialty boards, which examine each candidate.

Thus, a professor of surgery at a university might be the director of his own residency program; a member of the American Board of Surgery, which examines the graduates of his program; and a member of the residency review committee, which approves the residency programs and is organized under the joint aegis of the American Board of Surgery and the AMA's Council on Medical Education.

Such an oligarchy had the potential for almost unlimited power. It could have limited the number of physicians it would admit to its specialty by controlling the number of residency positions. In cooperation with similar oligarchies in other specialties, it could have set fees and established closed shops in the nation's hospitals. But it never did. On the contrary, the specialties have evidenced a strong belief in the free enterprise system, with each taking a laissez-faire attitude toward the affairs of other specialties. Certainly there was, and still is, some bickering over turf in particular areas of specialization. For instance, which specialist should perform head and neck surgery for cancer—the cancer surgeon, the nose and throat specialist, or the oral surgeon? And the association of all the specialists, the American Board of Medical Specialty Societies, has tended to be more concerned with internecine matters than with how the specialties can cooperate to provide needed care for the American public.

In retrospect, the various specialties and organized medicine in general, and especially the AMA, should have been as concerned with their responsibility to the public as they were with the autonomy of the profession. They should have developed a way of balancing the supply of specialists with the need—before the situation got out of hand.* Freedom without responsibility usually leads to anarchy and the development of specialization of medical practice, in America was no exception.

Unfortunately, in the formative years, the directors of residency programs seemed motivated to enlarge the size and, presumably, the prestige of their own programs. In other words, the number of residents was controlled, not by the needs of the American public, but the needs of the program and its director. Nor did the residency review committees provide a check. As long as there was sufficient "clinical material" available to provide each resident with a well-rounded educational experience, they approved the program.

Cost was no barrier to the size of a residency program. The expense was simply passed on to the consumer, the patient, as an allowable cost of hospital care.

The inclusion of residency costs was not without warrant. The resident-in-training was providing patient care services in exchange for his or her education. The charge, however, did not appear on the hospital bill as a separate item; it was hidden in the price of room and board, with all the other overhead costs. This deception was not deliberate; the best financial analysts have been unable to agree on how to identify the costs of medical education and balance them against the value of services the residents provide.

The only thing we can be sure of is that the cost has increased markedly over the years. In 1950, a resident in the most sought-after residency was paid $25 per month, or $300 per year. In 1970, a resident's salary ranged from $10,000 to $15,000 per year, a 5,000% increase over a period when inflation alone (at 6% per year) would have increased it by only 120%. The rising cost of medical education helps to explain why an appendectomy will now cost more in a teaching hospital than in a nonteaching hospital in the same community. Whether the care is better and therefore worth more depends on many factors.

Other reasons for the increased specialization in medical practice could be cited, such as the lure of more regular and shorter working hours and the potential for greater income. But whatever the cause, the point is: *The*

---

* In 1973, based on the Millis Commission report on graduate medical education, an attempt to control specialization was made. But this effort came rather late. Only now, ten years later, are we beginning to see some reduction in the number of residencies. The organization established in 1973 was the Liaison Committee on Graduate Medical Education—its name recently changed to Accreditation Council on Graduate Medical Education (ACGME)—representing all specialties, the hospitals, the medical schools, the AMA, the government, and the consumers. This organization has the capability to eventually control the numbers, types, and proportion of graduate medical education programs and, indirectly, the profile of physicians in practice.

magnitude of the move by physicians into specialized practice has not been based on the medical care needs of the American public but on the needs and desires of the profession.

Of course the profession needed to specialize as knowledge and technology increased. But it failed to control the numbers, types, and distribution of specialists in relation to medical care needs. What we have now is a mismatched system of medical care, in which 80% of physicians are specialists when only 20% are needed, and only 20% of physicians are trained and interested in providing primary care when 80% are needed.

Analyses of patient-physician encounters have repeatedly shown that 80% of all encounters require only the knowledge and skills of a general practitioner. But in our disproportionate system, 60% of encounters unnecessarily utilize the knowledge and skills—and the thinking—of a specialist. The result is usually that the patient receives poor care at a high cost. That is, the patient is frequently overtreated and has to pay the high fee of a specialist. Take Joe's ingrown toenail, for example.

❧ Joe can't resist a sale on one-size-fits-all socks at Macy's. But the socks are too short for his twelve-inch feet, and now he is suffering from an ingrown toenail. Since he doesn't have a family doctor, he goes to see his wife's internist.

The internist hasn't seen an ingrown toenail since he worked in the clinic as a resident. But he knows all about diabetes and its association with chronic infection.

"Joe," he says, "I don't think you have diabetes. But let's make sure you don't. You didn't mention any family history of the disease in the questionnaire you filled out while you were waiting, but that's not always necessary. Do you find cuts and scrapes take a long time to heal?"

"I don't know. How long is long?"

"More than a couple of weeks."

"No. I don't think so, anyway."

"Well, let's not take any chances. I want you to have a glucose tolerance test at the hospital tomorrow morning. We'll also get some basic lab tests, just to establish a baseline. And while you're there you might as well stop in X ray and get a chest film. I see you haven't had one in two years. My nurse will give you all the instructions. Good-bye."

"What about my toe?"

"Oh, just soak it in some warm water, morning and night. And keep a bandage on it."

A week later, Joe receives a phone call from the internist. The same day he receives a bill from the hospital for over $200 in lab and X-ray fees, expenses his insurance won't cover because the tests were done on an outpatient basis and were all normal.

"Joe," says the internist, "glad to report you don't have diabetes. All your tests were normal and so was your chest X ray. Oh, by the way, how is your toe?"

"Still the same, Doc."

"Oh. Do you know any surgeons?"

"No."

"Well, there's a new young orthopedic surgeon in town. They say he's terrific on feet. Name is Ramsey. I'll have my nurse set up an appointment."

"What about a podiatrist?"

"Don't believe in them, Joe. You'd better see Dr. Ramsey."

Two months later, Joe's toenail has finally healed and he is able to wear his one-size-fits-all socks again. His experience has cost him over $500, and he complains to his boss that the company's health insurance hasn't covered anything—not the hospital bill, not the pharmacy bill, not the internist's fee, not the surgeon's fee. Nothing.

"Joe," advises his boss, "next time try my family doctor. I had an ingrown toenail last year. He just put some cotton under it, cut a V in the nail, and told me my socks were too short. It healed in a couple of weeks and didn't cost me more than ten bucks." ❧

CHAPTER 6

Enter Government:
The Seeds of Destruction

PERHAPS it was inevitable that while we were creating the golden age of medicine we were inadvertently planting seeds for its potential destruction. Has it always been so? Was the writer of Ecclesiastes correct?

> To everything there is a season,
> And a time for every purpose under the heaven:
> A time to be born, and a time to die;
> A time to plant, and a time to pluck up that which is planted;
> A time to kill, and a time to heal;
> A time to break down, and a time to build up . . .

There were no villains plotting the destruction of the medical care system just as its golden age was being proclaimed. There was no conspiracy. All thought they were doing the right thing. They were simply carried away, swept up by their own success. Only now, in retrospect, do the sins of omission stand out so clearly.

Again, the move to specialization proves a telling example of how good intentions may lead to unexpected and undesirable results. Without question, specialization was necessary, and individual physicians sincerely believed that by specializing they could bring more knowledge to bear in treating their patients. But these specialists could no longer take care of all of a patient's needs; they no longer had the knowledge to serve as the physician of first contact when a patient became ill, to provide primary care.

Care became fragmented. Patients now had to go to several physicians to receive the spectrum of services formerly provided by a single general practitioner. The specialists, focused on their chosen field, were less concerned with the general health of their patients than with their particular illnesses. Moreover, as knowledge in their chosen areas increased, specialists found they knew more and more about less and less. They were soon isolated and lost sight of the larger picture. They were unaware of what was happening to the health care system. And profound changes were taking place.

Suddenly, the status of medical care shifted. Historically, medical attention had been a privilege of the affluent; they could afford to have a physician hold their hand when they were sick, or minister to their emotional needs, or provide the latest and most fashionable "cure." It had made little or no difference in most illnesses whether a physician was in attendance or not. Indeed, the poor and uneducated often felt they were better off without a doctor. But now it *did* make a difference whether or not one had access to a physician. One's life might depend on it. It had become a necessity.

The golden age of medicine did not go unnoticed by the poor and the underserviced minorities. They might not have access to medical care, but most had access to a TV set, and they wanted the kind of care they saw Dr. Kildare and Dr. Marcus Welby providing.

The civil rights movement of the 1950s became their voice, and the politicians heard their demands. The American Medical Association continued to argue that no one in the U.S. was ever denied needed care, that physicians always provided free care to those who could not pay. But this stance was no longer viable. The poor and minorities no longer wanted charity. Medical care was a right, and they demanded equal access.

Politicians became interested in health and the health status of Americans in relation to people in other nations. They looked at access to medical care in a different light. They saw it as a necessity that could and should be regulated by government just like any other utility. Soon, the issue of medical care became a political football, to be tossed around anew with each election. National health insurance and even socialized medicine appeared to be excellent topics for debate. And it was easier to play with this football in a climate of crisis, so the 'crisis' in American health care was created by political clamor in the midst of our golden age.

Politicians equated lack of access with an inadequate number of physicians. They demanded that we expand our medical schools. The AMA countered that no shortage of physicians existed. So throughout most of the Cold War, a hotter war was waged between the AMA and the federal government as to which was right. The government accused the AMA of trying to control the supply of physicians for economic reasons by restricting the number and size of the medical schools. The AMA charged the government with interfering in the practice of medicine.

They were both right. There probably was no shortage in the total number of physicians but a relative shortage existed because of the maldistribution of physicians brought on by the move into specialization. The problem of a sudden and marked decrease in the number of primary care physicians was compounded by poor geographic distribution.

The division of labor involved in specialization made it necessary for physicians to work in centers where cross-referral could easily occur. Specialists moved from the inner cities and rural areas to the suburbs, where there were more doctors and more affluent patients. They occupied offices in the same buildings, usually near a hospital. But they did not, as yet, form group practices. This was still frowned on by the AMA.

Attempts by specialists to join together in groups to provide primary care were continually rebuffed by the AMA. One apparent reason for this rejection was that some of the earliest and most enterprising groups were formed in association with prepayment plans. "Contract medicine" was still a dirty phrase. Had the AMA not taken this stand, perhaps the transition to specialization would have been smoother and the "shortage" corrected.

The government proceeded with a series of initiatives to improve access to medical care services. Through various grant programs, it tried to increase the number of physicians being trained. At the same time it began to provide payment for medical care for those who could not afford it. Although the government had previously provided direct medical care for the merchant marine, native Americans, and the armed forces, this was the first time it had entered the private sector of the medical marketplace to purchase care.

The Kerr-Mills Act of 1962 provided funds for the care of the indigent aged. The Health Professions Educational Assistance Act of 1963 provided construction funds and capitation grants to encourage medical schools to increase the size of their classes. Public Law (P.L.) 89–290, enacted in 1964, created medical scholarships and supplied funds to support the operating costs for the schools, beyond the NIH grants.

Then, in 1965, Congress approved the Medicare and Medicaid amendments to the Social Security Act (P.L. 89–97). With this legislation, Congress declared that a minimum level of health care was the right of every U.S. citizen. The law provided financing for health care services for the elderly (Medicare) and for the poor (Medicaid). Medicare, through an intermediary (usually Blue Cross), provided direct payment for care of the elderly individual. Under the Medicaid program, grants for medical care were given to the states to administer under their individual welfare systems. (The federal government paid at least 50% of a state's budget for these services. Benefits in the Medicaid program varied from state to state, depending on the individual state's "wealth.") Thus, overnight the government had become the largest single purchaser of medical care.

As might have been anticipated, Medicare and Medicaid compounded the shortage problem by increasing the demand for services. The physician shortage was particularly evident in hospital care, especially teaching hospitals, because the poor and the elderly utilized these services to a greater extent than did the rest of the population. Again, the shortage appeared more acute than it really was, especially with the push to set up more residency programs.

Residency positions were created faster than the medical schools could graduate M.D.'s to fill them. Many positions remained vacant, and the hospitals and government began to look to other sources for house staff. Graduates of foreign medical schools, often eager to train in the United States, offered an easy solution—it would be much faster to hire them than to wait for American medical schools to enlarge their enrollment. The State Department cooperated by lifting the immigration quotas for physicians, and America was flooded with foreign medical graduates.

Many of these foreign physicians were well qualified, but others were not. Some could not speak or understand the English language and thus could not really benefit from the educational opportunity. The Educational Commission for Foreign Medical Graduates was eventually established to set language and educational standards and to screen applicants from abroad. Although the standards for admission to the graduate medical education programs were raised, many problems still existed.

In fact, this "solution" to the physician "shortage" created more problems than it solved. On the surface, the concept looked good—in addition to filling residency slots, we could share our know-how by training many of the world's physicians. But it didn't work out that way. Our graduate education residencies were designed to teach the individual physician to practice in the United States. They operated under the assumption that the resources, especially the technology, available to the trained physicians in America would also be available in other countries. Except in Europe, this was not the case. Foreign physicians often found their newly acquired knowledge and skills worthless in their own country. The tools they had learned to use were not available. Disillusioned, many decided to practice here instead of returning home. Others intentionally used their education as their passport for immigration. Many married American citizens and acquired citizenship through their spouse.

The result was a great brain drain to America from the developing countries of the Third World. India and the Philippines were affected most; together, they supplied 30% of all foreign medical graduates in the 1960s. The total numbers increased each year.

In 1972, 46% of all new licenses to practice medicine were given to foreign medical graduates. Although the annual number has decreased since that time, in 1978 the percentage was still 23.6%. By the end of 1978, there were 91,351 foreign medical graduates in the United States, accounting for 20.9% of the total physician population. Of the foreign medical graduates, only 9.5% engaged in general practice; the rest became specialists, thus adding to the problem of overspecialization.

Some foreign medical students, unable to pass the examinations necessary for full licensure, have been exploited by being granted limited licenses to practice. In Illinois, for example, limited licenses restrict the graduate's practice to a hospital, theoretically under supervision. Yet most of these individuals are not qualified to practice medicine at all, and the care they provide in mental and other state-run hospitals is substandard. The policy of limited licensure should be condemned.

It is important to remember that many individual foreign medical graduates have made outstanding contributions to American medicine over the years, and they have become valuable U.S. citizens. Nevertheless, the rapid influx of such a large number over a relatively short period of time highlighted certain difficulties in cultural assimilation. Many foreign students did not mix socially with Americans; instead, they tended to stay together and continued to speak to one another in their native tongue. This isolation not only fostered the language barrier in communicating with other doctors and patients, but it also perpetuated cultural differences. A native of the Philippines, for example, has a much different approach to pain than someone raised in the United States. Philippine culture teaches one to ignore pain and to bear it without complaint. But the Philippine doctor who ignores an American patient's complaints of pain might appear insensitive.

Paradoxically, while we were easing the standards for admission to residency programs and subsequently to practice in the United States, we were tightening the standards for admission to our own medical schools. As a consequence, many qualified Americans were denied the right to choose the practice of medicine as their lifework. Although the size of American schools nearly doubled and many new schools were opened, the tightened standards actually decreased the opportunity for admission for many people-oriented individuals who would have become excellent general practitioners.

As a result, the character of the American physician also changed with the new standards for admission to medical school. "Only eggheads need apply" became the guiding principle of admission committees. Although most schools claimed they gave equal consideration to three criteria—college grade point average, score on the standard medical aptitude test, and the personal interview—in reality, unless an applicant's college grade point average was above 3.8 (out of a possible 4.0), he or she received no further consideration. Apparently, the individual's motivation or character, essential factors in any service profession, did not count. Perhaps it was because the new physicians were all specialists, and the emphasis was on knowledge and technology, that personal characteristics were overlooked.

Unfortunately, the change in admission criteria occurred at a time when applications to medical schools were increasing. No longer did medical students have to struggle, borrow money, put off marriage until after they began practice. They could get government grants for their tuition or guaranteed loans—which they could pay back in a year or two on a specialist's income—and they could support a family on a resident's salary of $15,000 plus room and board. Competition for admission to medical school became a vicious game with no holds barred—an experience that would better qualify one to become an officer of the Green Berets than a family doctor in Hometown, U.S.A. Take the case of Jimmy Smith, for example.

⊷§ Jimmy Smith lives next door. All his life, Jimmy has wanted to be a doctor. I remember that when he was in high school he couldn't learn enough about biology. He would bring over his collection of insects and, later, his dissections of frogs and lampreys to show me. In his senior year, after football season was over (he was the quarterback on our local high school team), I arranged for him to spend his Saturdays in the anatomy lab at the medical school in town.

Two nights a week Jimmy worked as a volunteer at Beverly House, the nursing unit attached to the Old Folks Home. He would give bed baths to some of the older men, act as an orderly, and read to those who couldn't see to read for themselves. The excitement that shone in his eyes when he recounted these experiences always touched me. I'll never forget his telling me about the death of one old man while he held his hand—but that is something special between Jim and me.

Jim decides not to play football in college. "I'm pretty small compared to the size of some of these guys, and besides, I want to concentrate on my studies," he writes in a letter. Jim is bright and intelligent, but he has to work for his grades. Math is his downfall. He flunks one calculus course and, even though he wins honors in history, his grade point average is only 2.98. It isn't enough for medical school.

"I'm pretty discouraged," he writes. "The competition is fierce. The ten guys and two girls in my class who have been admitted to med school so far are all 'egg heads.' They all have a grade point average of 3.9 or better. Three of them even have a straight 4.0. But none of them gives a damn about people. Two of these guys cheated on their exams all through school. And one—we all know it but can't prove it—sabotaged my best friend's final lab experiment in organic chemistry, just to get the highest grade in the course.

"My mother says that if that's the kind of person they are admitting to medical school these days, I'd be better off going into some other field. At times, I think she's right. But I'm not willing to give up yet, even if it doesn't look too good. My friend and I are taking Spanish this year with the idea that we might apply to Guadalajara in Mexico, if we can't get into an American school. Fifteen from last year's premed class went there.

"I haven't heard yet from your school. Anything you can do to help me, I'd certainly appreciate."

I call the dean of admissions the next day.

"Joe," I ask, "where does James Smith's application stand?"

"The admissions committee turned him down early this week. I guess he hasn't received his notification yet."

"No!" I am more than angry. I am furious. "Son of a bitch!"

"Sorry, Tom," he says. "Your letter really moved the committee. They had a hard time turning him down after reading it. But you know how it is. We're a state university, and all sorts of people scrutinize what we do. We can't show any favoritism. You have no idea how much pressure is put on us from all sides. The governor is always on the phone. The only way we can survive is to stick strictly to our criteria."

"Damn it! I didn't ask for any favors. That boy would have made an excellent doctor. You'd better look at your criteria."

"I know. I know. These are funny times. There was just no way we could take him unless he had a 3.8 average."

"I thought you were giving priority to those who want to go into general practice. This boy wants to be a family doctor."

"We're more concerned with *where* they will practice. We have to look at their background and try to pick those likely to practice in the inner city, among their own . . . or out in the sticks."

"What about this Guadalajara medical school? Jim's thinking about going there."

"It's certainly not the best solution in the world. The classes are huge—over a thousand. Also, the lectures are given in Spanish, so he'd need to know the language. And they don't get any lab experience. Yet some Americans make it going there. We have a couple here as residents who are going to make excellent physicians—they're so highly motivated, they put some of our own graduates to shame. I suppose if he wants to be a doctor bad enough, he'll go to any extreme. Tom, let me level with you. You and I probably couldn't get into medical school today if we tried."

"Thanks," I say and hang up. "And you'll know where to shove that next request for money," I yell into the dead mouthpiece. It doesn't help. ๕๛

CHAPTER 7

The Height of the Golden Age:
A Time of "Crisis"

PHYSICIANS thought it ludicrous that America's golden age of medicine should also be labeled "a time of crisis in health care" by politicians. Didn't they realize that during the 1950s and 1960s we had accomplished more than in all of history in the treatment of disease? Infectious diseases were under control; we would never again suffer from the plagues and pestilence of the past.

Physicians most resented being held responsible for deficiencies in the health of our citizens and for the United States' low rating, compared with other countries, on such measures as infant mortality. But it seemed to be politically expedient to blame the medical profession, even when the real causes were unemployment, hunger, poor housing, and lack of education—problems more easily solved by the politician than the physician.

Most physicians would freely admit that they believed their responsibility involved the diagnosis and treatment of disease only, not the preservation and restoration of health. Health promotion and the prevention of disease, in their opinion, were the responsibility of the public health field, not of medicine. Just keeping abreast of all the new breakthroughs in the treatment of disease during this golden age was more than enough to consume all a physician's time and effort.

"Actually," asserted the American Medical Association in the profession's defense, "we wouldn't appear so bad if politicians would stop comparing the entire United States with some Scandinavian country [the Scandinavian countries usually had the best health indices]. Scandinavia doesn't have our Harlems and Wattses. If you compare Norway or Sweden with the state of Minnesota—places with a similar climate, size, and ethnic makeup—Minnesota rates just as high."

"But we spend more per capita on health care than any other country," protested the politicians. "Why aren't our statistics better?" But here they were confused. We were spending more per capita on *medical care*, not health care. In the late 1960s, 98% of our "health" budget went

55

to the treatment of illness; only 2% was used for the promotion of health and the prevention of disease.

The cry of a "critical shortage of physicians" was also mostly political. It was a case of misdiagnosis and the treatment became a case of mismanagement. As we have said, the problem was really poor distribution —too many physicians in specialties and not enough in primary care, too great a concentration of physicians in the suburbs and not enough in the inner cities and rural areas. To solve this problem simply by trying to increase the total number of physicians—without addressing the problem of distribution—was poor judgment. It would lead to a "surplus" of physicians within twenty years.

The poor lived in areas that had always been underserved by physicians. Many were minorities who lived in the inner cities, the Harlems and the Wattses. Others lived in sparsely populated areas of rural America, like Appalachia. Yet it wasn't simply the lack of payment that had kept physicians from moving into these areas in the past. The promise of payment wasn't going to suddenly solve the problem. Nor did the purposeful selection of medical students from these areas, with the hope they would return home to practice, work. Still, for a time it seemed as if there might be a solution.

Under the impetus of the social revolution that swept across America in the 1960s, the whole appearance of the young doctor changed. He wore blue jeans, open-toed sandals, and a T-shirt with his white coat; his hair was long and he grew a beard. She wore loose shifts, no bra, and her hair hung straight down to her waist. These young physicians moved to the inner cities and rural areas to set up practice. Soon, however, they had children of school age (many had started to raise families in medical school). Then, one by one, the men shaved their beards and the women put on bras, and they moved with their families to affluent suburbia. It wasn't that they weren't motivated anymore, but the seemingly unsolvable problems of poverty-stricken neighborhoods, the desires of their spouses, and the concern for their children proved to be the dominating influences.

The problem of geographic distribution is not unique to a free enterprise system of medical care. Most of the countries that have socialized medical care—Sweden, for example—have the same problem. In the United States, it is the hospital that has offered a partial solution. In the inner cities, the clinics of the teaching hospitals—purposely located in these areas—have long served as the primary source of medical care for the poor. The nation's first hospital, the Pennsylvania Hospital in Philadelphia, is a typical example.

Moreover, some of the large public hospitals, such as Boston City, Bellevue in New York, Charity in New Orleans, Cook County in Chicago, and San Francisco General, are among the best hospitals in the country. I always tell my friends that if they are ever in an accident or become ill in New York City, they should ask to be taken to Bellevue. They couldn't find better care. The amenities may be scarce, but the care is good. And even though Marcus Welby doesn't practice there, some of the resident physicians closely resemble young Dr. Kildare.

Hospitals also provide rural America with primary and emergency care. Half of the 7,000 hospitals in the United States are under a hundred beds in size, and many of these are in otherwise underserviced locations. The Hill-Burton Law of 1946 allowed local communities to build their own hospitals by guaranteeing low-interest loans and grants (up to two-thirds the cost of construction). As a result, most communities have a hospital within thirty-five miles. While many of these institutions are not fully staffed, most Americans at least have access to emergency services, given modern communication and transportation networks.

Although hospitals per se cannot practice medicine (diagnosis and treatment) and they do not automatically come equipped with a medical staff, they do attract physicians to a community. They also serve as the site of employment of nonphysician members of the health care team: nurses, physician assistants, and technicians. New and innovative arrangements for the delivery of health care services, using a team approach, have been tried in these settings to provide more care with fewer physicians.

American ingenuity was much in evidence during the period of debate over the physician "shortage." The use of allied health professionals, especially the idea of converting former medical corpsmen in the armed forces into civilian counterparts, received major emphasis. New health professionals—physician assistants, nurse-midwives, and pediatric nurse-practitioners—were encouraged and were even permitted some degree of independent practice under the supervision of a physician.

Most of these innovative experiments, however, were just that—experiments. There was no clear effort to identify the real problems or to work out a plan for their solution. And many of the answers later turned up as new problems. The approach was piecemeal. The United States had no national health policy.

If one had asked the average American physician during the late 1960s whether we needed a national health policy, the response would probably have been a quizzical look and a quick dismissal—"I'm too busy to think about that." Most physicians lived and worked in affluent suburbia and, from the perspective there, they probably did not see the changes brought about by specialization. They were unaware that for a growing number of people access was a problem; it wasn't evident in their practice. What stood out for these physicians was the increase in knowledge and technology, discoveries that made it possible to do more and more for their patients.

Even if one had explained the problems, one probably would have heard the same kind of reassurance these physicians constantly gave their patients. "It's a necessary trade-off for all the progress we're making. It's inconvenient, but it's a temporary bother, one that will adjust itself, given enough time, in our free enterprise system."

ᥱ§ It is 1970, and John Cleaver, M.D., F.A.C.S., is now 55 years old. He is chief of surgery at Community Hospital and teaches at the university, where he is associate clinical professor of surgery. (Clinical professor is the title reserved for the voluntary faculty, those that teach part-time without being paid.) Cleaver enjoys teaching and is proud that the university sends its third- and forth-year residents to rotate on his service for part of their training. One of these residents, Bob Stewart, is closing a case for him now. Cleaver left the operating room so that Stewart would know that he trusted him and had confidence in his skill and judgment.

"Thank you, Lord, for helping with this case," he murmurs under his breath as he strips off his gloves and lights a cigarette. He always prays before and after each operation, just as he always reviews the anatomy in the classic text *Gray's Anatomy* before each procedure and immediately dictates his operation report at the conclusion. No one knows he prays, but people do know he is an elder of the First Presbyterian Church.

They also know he lives in a $150,000 home in the best part of town and that he married Marsha Johnson, a pretty student nurse he met thirty years ago in this very hospital, when he was a medical student. Some say he did and others said he didn't know her father was president of the First National Bank when he first started dating her. (She lived in the nurses' home.) In any case, her father was furious when they eloped on December 8, 1941, and a week after their marriage John went off to war as a medical officer and Marsha came back to finish her nurse's training. But Marsha's father stopped being angry when, on September 14, 1942, John Cleaver, Jr., was born in Community Hospital.

Everyone knows that Dr. Cleaver was wounded at Anzio in January

1944 and came home a war hero, with a stainless steel kneecap in his left leg.

"That's why he drives an MG—to keep his knee 'in shape.' "

"And you would have thought that Dr. Cleaver was old Mr. Johnson's own son, the way he bragged about Dr. Cleaver's getting that prized residency in surgery at the university . . . and building that house for them and all, while Dr. Cleaver was still a resident."

"Yes. Dr. Cleaver certainly has it made."

"But it couldn't have happened to a nicer guy."

"Big house, happy marriage, three cars. . . ."

"Still, he's one of the few doctors that always remembers your name."

"And he's real friendly."

"By the way, did you know that his hands are insured for a million dollars?"

While Cleaver is aware that the nurses talk about him like this, he would be embarrassed and surprised to know that he is the subject of similar conversations over the back fence, on the telephone, all over town. His surgical successes are embroidered with each telling, and his failures are never mentioned. People have confidence in Dr. Cleaver. He is a symbol of the golden age of medicine. Yet Cleaver is aware of the terrible responsibility that comes with power and authority.

It has been a long operation and he is tired. His knee aches and he rubs it unconsciously. It is good to sit in this leather chair in the doctor's lounge and drink his coffee and smoke. It relaxes him. He looks at his hands, still covered with the starch powder that absorbed his sweat and caked under his gloves.

To think, he says to himself, that a few minutes ago these hands held a living human heart. Imagine being able to stop a heart while one operates on it, replace a damaged mitral valve with an artificial one, close the heart, and then start it again. John Cleaver has never stopped being amazed at what he can now do as a result of the fantastic advances in medical knowledge and technology. It seems as though each week brings another new breakthrough that makes his work more successful and safer, allowing him to do more and more.

Years before it happened, he knew that someone would find out how to transplant the human heart. So he was not surprised when, in 1967, Christiaan Barnard of South Africa performed the first successful heart transplant. It was just a matter of time after John Gibbon at Jefferson performed the first open heart operation, with the aid of his heart-lung machine, in 1953. Cleaver had seen that first machine of John's. How crude it was compared with the one they had used this morning!

He remembers the agony of arriving at a decision to do open heart surgery in this hospital. He had just been made chief when the issue came up, and he was imbued with a new sense of responsibility. He felt torn between the challenge to do it—he was personally excited by the idea—and the size of the projected cost ($26,000 a case, the administrator calculated). The cardiologists on the staff exerted the most pressure; they didn't want to lose their patients by having to transfer them to University Hospital for open heart surgery. They cornered the chairman of the hospital's board of trustees in the locker room of the golf club and pressed their case. The chairman was told that doing open heart surgery would raise the prestige of Community Hospital.

The next day, Cleaver received a phone call from the board chairman.

"John, I understand the staff's executive committee at its next meeting is going to discuss the possibility of doing open heart surgery. I just wanted you to know that the board will be receptive to the idea, if you want to push for it. It will be your decision, however. You doctors know best."

Had it been a wise decision, even with the board underwriting the cost? The decision raised his own income by well over $100,000 a year, but the hospital was still only just breaking even. When he voiced his feelings of guilt about this and offered to personally make up any loss the hospital sustained, the administrator informed him that the revenues from the cardiologists' catheterization lab were more than covering the loss. He was glad he didn't know too much about hospital economics—best to leave that to the administrator and the board.

But he put his foot down when the young Turks wanted to do kidney transplants. Like the cardiologists, the dialysis boys—his pet name for the three nephrologists on the staff—complained of having to transfer all their end-stage renal disease patients to University Hospital. They, too, bypassed him and went directly to the board, but by this time Cleaver was director of the whole surgical department and a much better politician.

Again, he received a phone call from the chairman of the board, but he told him right out that transplant surgery was too complicated and expensive for a community hospital. Furthermore, if the board wanted the continued prestige of a university affiliation, it had better understand that the university expected us to refer all our organ transplant patients to the professor of surgery at University Hospital. Our affiliation was a matter of give and take; we needed the residents the university sent to us.

"Understand perfectly, John," said the chairman. "You stick to your guns; we'll back you up."

The board wasn't too happy, however, when the nephrologists moved out of the hospital and set up their own freestanding kidney dialysis unit across the street. Cleaver explained to the board that in the long run the university affiliation was more important to the hospital. But the nephrologists became millionaires in about two years, and the hospital lost all that revenue.

Thinking about it now, Cleaver still believes he was right. Even today, transplants are far from being routinely successful. Admittedly, immunologists did achieve a major breakthrough when they learned how to delay and attenuate the body's rejection of a foreign organ from another person—a phenomenon that made the early transplant operations so difficult. We now know how to type and cross–match tissues, just as we do with blood. And there are new drugs that inhibit the body's immune responses in order to prevent rejection of a transplant.

Still, preventing rejection is a continuous battle. After all, as a species, we owe our selection for survival in large part to the immune response to foreign substances. It has taken uncounted millennia to program the defense against a hostile environment into our genes. It is this individualized defense that makes each of us so unique, Cleaver muses. I doubt it can ever be totally overpowered, although scientists are certainly making the attempt.

His reverie is interrupted as Bob Stewart comes into the lounge, a cup of coffee in one hand and the patient's chart in the other.

"How did it go? Any trouble in closing?"

"No, sir. Everything went fine. Would you like to check these orders?"

Cleaver reads the order sheet and nods his approval. "You might ask Dr. Dilworth, the patient's internist, if he agrees with the insulin regimen you have set up. He'll probably let you handle it. But, out of courtesy, I'd ask him."

"Certainly. I'll call him from the recovery room. I want to go in there and check on the mechanical ventilator settings," Stewart replies over his shoulder as he hurries out of the lounge.

"Let me know when everything has settled down. I want to bring his wife in to see him as soon as possible."

Cleaver knows how comforting it can be just to see a loved one, even for a moment, in the recovery room. He also knows how frightening it can be to see all those respirators, monitors, arterial and intravenous lines, with tubes sticking out of every orifice. That's why he wants everything settled down before he takes Mrs. Arnold in to see her husband. He has already stopped in the waiting room to assure her that all went well.

He himself is awed, if not frightened, by the technology that accompanies his profession these days. Certainly, he's grateful for the technicians and the medical subspecialists who know how to keep all those machines running. He has nightmares of being left alone in the intensive care unit. Suddenly, the alarms on all the monitors begin to ring at once, and the nurses and technicians are all off on a coffee break. He wakes up in a cold sweat.

Marsha has been after him to take a year off for a sabbatical, now that the kids are out of college. "Your father took one every seven years," she keeps reminding him.

"But he was a history professor. History doesn't change that fast. If I took a year off, I'd be so far behind I'd never catch up. It's all I can do to keep up, let alone catch up. I wouldn't dare."

He knows that the ground he works won't stay fallow for a year. And he knows there are those that will delight in plowing his practice under should he be away that long. No, he doesn't dare.

There are compensations, however. Like this morning. When a case goes well, he experiences the glow of euphoria, the satisfaction of a job well done. It always brings to mind the best moments of his life in this profession he dearly loves. He treasures those memories and feels it is important to share them with the students he teaches. A sense of history, his father would say, makes you appreciate the present. Now he knows what the old man meant.

Take Mr. Arnold, the man he just operated on, a diabetic. Before 1921, when Frederick G. Banting and Charles H. Best discovered insulin, diabetes was incurable. Today Mr. Arnold can be operated on safely, and he'll probably live another ten years. Endocrinology—Cleaver reflects—a new specialty in my lifetime. Cortisone. I hope Mr. Arnold won't need it, but it's nice to have on hand if a patient goes into shock or develops an allergy to some medication. And the *pill*, what would women do without it, or men, too, for that matter. He smiles. A diaphragm didn't prevent John Jr.

And the vitamins and minerals in the intravenous solutions—the young doctors today take them for granted. The first time he added potassium to an IV, the pathologist yelled at him over the phone: "What are you trying to do, kill your patient?" He ended up taking reprints from the journals down to the pathologist's office and showing him all about potassium metabolism, how a deficiency occurs in surgical patients and can suddenly stop the heart. It was hard to keep up on everything in those days, too. And *Future Shock* hadn't even been written.

Nutrition. How important it is. Only now are they even beginning to teach it in medical school. And improved nutrition has had more effect in controlling infectious diseases than all the antibiotics we have developed. True, the effect of good nutrition is slower, less spectacular, but it's more lasting because it increases the body's resistance to disease.

Antibiotics. It's hard to recall practicing without them. But they, too, were discovered in his lifetime. He wouldn't think of putting an artificial valve into a heart, as he had done this morning, without having prophylactic antibiotics available to prevent possible infection. Penicillin was the big one. He remembered when it first came out . . . when it had to be given IV . . . that was when he was in North Africa. Penicillin had probably saved his life when that mortar tore up his knee at Anzio. That and tetanus toxoid.

But immunology, with its focus on increasing the body's resistance to infection, was probably going to be more important than all the antibiotics. It probably holds the key to our conquest of cancer. We know now that cancer is many separate diseases, not one. And there are many factors, not one, that cause it. Perhaps the most important factor is host resistance—and that may depend on immunity. We'll prevent cancer, Cleaver speculates, before we learn to cure it.

"Mr. Arnold is awake and asking for you, Doctor." Bob Stewart sticks his head in the doorway. "He was fighting the respirator, so I discontinued it."

"Thanks, Bob. Wait, I'll come with you."

As they walk down the hall together, Cleaver puts his hand on the younger man's shoulder. "Bob," he says, "we're lucky men to be practicing our profession in a golden age. I've been thinking about all the incredible advances in my lifetime. For all those discoveries to be made, there had to be the freedom to experiment, the drive to leave the world better than we found it. None of it would have been possible without our free enterprise system of medical care." ❧

CHAPTER 8

The War Is On: Family Practice Becomes a Specialty

WHAT the John Cleavers of American medicine didn't realize was that by 1970 we no longer had a free enterprise system of medical care.

We began to erode the medical marketplace in the 1930s when we used Blue Cross prepayment plans to finance hospital care. The cost reimbursement tactic was our first mistake. And it was compounded by direct payment to providers by the plans that placed a third party between the provider and the consumer (see Chapter 4). Consumers could no longer be prudent buyers. They had no idea what the care they needed would cost. Nor were they concerned—whatever it cost, they were covered.

Had this method of financing been confined to the private sector, where there was competition from the indemnity type of health insurance written by the commercial companies, we might have retained a semblance of a marketplace. But in 1965, we completely destroyed it by adopting the same financing mechanisms for Medicare and Medicaid—cost reimbursement of hospitals by an intermediary placed between the provider and the purchaser of care. Government had become the largest purchaser of care, and, unlike other consumers, it had the power to legislate. When the providers failed to meet its needs or desires, it simply legislated an increase in the supply side to meet its demands.

During the last half of the 1960s, government was responsible for stimulating an unprecedented increase in the number of physicians (foreign and domestic vintages), allied health professionals, hospital beds, the latest technology, and *health care costs.*

By 1970, however, the government had become concerned with the cost of health care, a cost it had generated, and a liberal Congress was spurred by the first conservative administration in years to do something about it. During the Nixon, Ford, and Carter administrations, the government tried, without success, to control—through regulation—the cost acceleration it had created. But the brakes didn't hold because no fundamental changes were made in the basic causes of the rising costs. The cost reimbursement mechanism, in particular, was left untouched.

Behind the scenes, however, a few members of the medical profession were trying to change another basic factor of the cost problem—overspecialization. The members of the American Academy of General Practice realized there was no correlation between the medical care system and the medical needs of the U.S. public. The academy was in trouble, as was American medicine, for the number of physicians in general practice had reached a new low of 17%. To offset the trend toward overspecialization, the academy put forward a brainchild of its own—the concept of family practice as a new specialty.

The new primary care physicians were to be different from the old general practitioners, although exhibiting the same tender loving care. They would no longer be "local medical doctors," at the bottom of the medical totem pole. They would be specialists, specialists in breadth if not in depth, but with the same status as other specialists. It was a matter of professional pride and morale.

These new specialists would be competent to handle 80% of all patient-physician encounters, and they would see that the other 20% got into the right hands. They would be qualified to act as primary care physicians for all members of the family, from the newborn—whom they could deliver—to the elderly. (Although, in line with the times, they would extend the definition of the family to include any living arrangement under one roof, even a single individual.) They would also be willing to work with allied health professionals in a team approach to care. The main emphasis, however, the guiding principle that separated family practice from other specialties, was the orientation to people rather than to a disease or organ system.

Except for the profession itself, this concept caught the imagination of nearly everyone concerned with the problem of overspecialization. The government saw it as the eventual answer to the problems of access, poor distribution, and the increasing cost of care. Congress responded with legislation to support the idea. The Comprehensive Health Manpower Training Act of 1971 (P.L. 92-157) provided funds for the development of departments of family practice in medical schools, as well as funds to increase the numbers of nonphysician health care providers.

Most of the medical profession, however, pleased with twenty years of increasing specialization, viewed this step as retrogressive. Pediatric and internal medicine specialists eyed it with horror. The pediatricians were alarmed because they already found themselves in oversupply and were extending their practice from children of six years to "children" of sixteen and even twenty-one. The internists saw a new phoenix rising from the ashes of general practice, a fire they thought they had put out once and for all. They gathered their extinguishers and girded themselves once more for battle. An internecine feud had begun.

◄§ Charlie is a gunfighter, a man of the Old West. Born in 1925 in Jackson, Wyoming, and raised in Colorado, on the eastern slopes of the Rockies, he is a cowboy, a hunter and trapper, a fly fisherman, a prospector, a philosopher, a historian, and a physician.

He started out as a general practitioner delivering babies, performing appendectomies and an occasional gallbladder operation, setting broken bones, and treating ingrown toenails. During the Korean War, he was both an anesthesiologist and a general surgeon in a MASH unit. Everything he does, he does well.

Charlie is as much at home delivering a baby in a one-room shack as dancing to a hot combo in the ballroom of the Brown Palace in Denver, and he dresses the same for both occasions. There are two things Charlie always wears—a grin and his Western boots with pointed toes. Even in the East.

Legend has it—Charlie became a legend to most of us—that he wears both of them to bed, and they were responsible for his reputation as a fantastic lover. I never had the courage to ask him about that, but he often talks about his boots whenever anyone looks down to see if he has them on.

"Always wear 'em," he'll explain. "Used to wear 'em for protection against rattlesnakes, but back East, here, they make good rat stabbers." Then he'll grin and walk away.

Charlie is one of the first to become board certified in the new specialty of family practice. By the time I meet him, he is the director of a family practice residency program in Denver. Charlie is a born teacher; he can identify with the students without becoming their peer.

I talk the dean of the medical school into bringing him East as a professor and chairman of the department of family practice. The dean has a fight on his hands. He needs a good gunfighter, and Charlie is the man for the job.

The dean doesn't like the term gunfighter, and every time I use it he corrects me. "Change agent," he says. "A change agent."

But I know he needs a gunfighter. I don't think he realizes how strong the feeling is against family practice or how bloody the battle is likely to become. He should—he's been trying for two years to get a department off the ground and he's already lost two men who tried to start it. One lasted almost a year, but the second gave up after only three months. He needs a gunfighter, someone who can stand up to Dr. Brown, the professor of internal medicine.

As the medical director of the hospital, I sit in on all the task force meetings on primary care. Eventually, it gets to be a broken record. I know everyone's stance by heart; I could write the minutes of a meeting before it takes place.

I play the devil's advocate at the meetings, a role assigned by the dean. I was a pulling guard in college football and now I'm playing that position again, protecting the quarterback. The dean is lying low. He knows the average life of a medical school dean is only two years, and he's in his third, living on borrowed time.

Dr. Brown always goes into the same speech at the beginning of our meetings. I guess he thinks if he repeats it often enough we'll all come to believe it.

"Internists," he proclaims, "are the new primary care physicians. We are the only specialists with the depth of knowledge to meet any need of a patient who comes seeking help. Years ago, before medicine was based on scientific knowledge, when frequently all a physician could do was to hold the patient's hand, general practitioners were useful. Now they're not; they don't know enough. If they had enough knowledge, they'd be internists."

"I agree with Dr. Brown," the chief of pediatrics invariably responds. "For adults, everything he says is right. But children have special needs only a pediatrician is trained to detect and treat."

I know that both of them constantly argue over the age at which jurisdiction should shift from the pediatrician to the internist, but in public they close ranks against the family physician.

"We are often the physician of first contact," the professor of obstetrics and gynecology interjects at some point, as though he were trying to justify his presence on a task force on primary care. Everyone ignores him.

"Remember," I remind them, "we are a tertiary care institution. We have a warped perspective of the real world. We see a very high proportion of really sick people, and we should. But the models we set up here for primary care should be the same as those our students are going to live with in their own practices. We do a beautiful job on secondary and tertiary care, but we are doing a lousy job of serving the primary care needs of our local community.

"We have to be the primary care physician for a neighborhood that extends for three miles on all sides of us. And what do we offer?

Only specialty clinics. These people don't need specialists; they need primary care. They are referred back and forth, from one clinic to another, and they rarely see the same doctor twice. Sometimes they have to wait a week for an appointment."

"They can always use the emergency room," interrupts Dr. Brown.

"No way," counters the chief of surgery, who is responsible for the professional aspects of the emergency room. "The ER is strictly for emergencies. My residents who staff it complain that people are using it as a source of general medical care. I tell them to refer all those people to the clinic."

"Do you know what it costs just to walk into our ER?" I ask. "I'll tell you—$45 before you see anyone."

"That's right," says the dean. "We constantly receive complaints from the community, from ministers and local politicians, that we are turning away too many people and that those we do treat can't afford our charges. We must establish a primary care clinic that will be open until at least 11:00 P.M. to meet the demand. That will also take the load off the emergency room. That's one reason I want a family practice program."

The same arguments seem to come up at each meeting, but the dean gradually makes some inroads. Internal medicine and pediatrics finally agree to a family practice outpatient clinic, but not inpatient service. Family practice physicians are to hospitalize their patients on either the medical or the pediatric service where they can be watched. The dean and I don't like it, but we take every little bit we can get. And this is where Charlie comes in; this is when I know we need a gunfighter.

Charlie makes quite an impression on the group—not all good, but not all bad either. Most of the chiefs seem to like Charlie right off. He makes the task force meetings more bearable, and they like the way he stands up to Dr. Brown. "Let's cut out the bullshit," Charlie says in a soft voice in the midst of one of Brown's tirades against family medicine. No one has ever seen the professor of internal medicine with his mouth open and nothing coming out; he shuts up for the rest of the meeting.

Charlie is always one jump ahead of them. He does his homework. I begin to look at it as a chess game. I try to figure out his strategy, when he'll make a new move here or there. It's like playing against a board of all kings and queens, no pawns. Charlie is just a knight, so he has to be fast on his feet. Every time he moves, he has to duck to one side or the other to keep his advantage. But soon he has them retreating to their ivory towers while he roams quite freely about the board, getting his job done. They have begun to respect him.

Take the shoot-out with the chief of obstetrics and gynecology, for example. It's the morning of our usual task force meeting, and by ten o'clock everyone knows that Charlie helped his own resident deliver a breech vaginally earlier that morning. Everything went well; both mother and baby are doing fine. But everyone also knows this is the first breech to be delivered normally in two years. There's a standing order from the chief that all breech presentations are to be delivered by Caesarean section. Charlie did stop in afterwards at the OB department office to explain the situation to the chief. But the chief's secretary informed Charlie that the chief couldn't see him that morning. Was he waiting to shoot Charlie down at the meeting, in front of an audience?

The task force meetings always take place at lunchtime; sandwiches and coffee are provided. The time, high noon, is probably the reason they call the meeting room the O.K. Corral.

The chief of obstetrics and gynecology fires the first shot. "Dr. Westward," he begins.

"Woodward," Charlie corrects him.

"Dr. Woodward," he starts again. "My resident informs me that one of your residents delivered a breech this morning, contrary to all the standing orders of my department."

"That's true, but under the circumstances . . ."

"There is a standing order that your residents are to ask for a consultation with my chief resident when any delivery is abnormal. And that includes malpresentations."

"My resident did call your resident, but your chief resident had never seen a breech delivered vaginally. He told my resident the patient would have to have a Caesarean section."

"That's right. That's my standing order."

"No exceptions?"

"No exceptions."

"What if the patient refuses?"

"Did this patient refuse?"

"No. She wasn't asked."

"You see," the chief says, looking around the room to be sure everyone is listening, "we cooperate with this man, let his residents use our delivery rooms, and what thanks do we get? He ignores our rules."

"She wasn't asked," Charlie continues, "because this was her fourth baby and the last two were breech presentations and were delivered normally. Hell, that little ass slipped out so smoothly you'd have thought it was a greased pig. No time to do a Caesarean, even though I can't understand why you would want to do one."

All eyes turn to the chief. He stammers, then recovers. "Be—because of the malpractice situation. If anything went wrong, and lots can go wrong with a breech, we'd be sitting ducks. I don't want to be on a witness stand with some smart-assed lawyer asking me why I didn't do a C-section."

Then, Charlie let him have the second barrel. "You could just as well be there explaining your 50% wound infection rate for your C-sections." Charlie really does his homework.

A year later Charlie resigns to take the chair in family practice at a western university, where he feels more at home—at least that's what he says. I suspect he got tired of the hassle, and there's no place here to go fishing on a bad day. In the eighteen months he was with us he accomplished a great deal.

He had set up a model family practice office right next to the emergency room. He used a team approach to primary care, with a nurse-practitioner, a medical social worker-educator, three residents (one from each year of training), and an attending physician who was actually in practice on each team. His program was fully accredited, and he made sure that his family practice program would survive by obtaining a three-year, $1-million grant to support it. Some of this money goes to other departments of the medical school that are willing to provide an educational rotation for the family practice residents on their services.

Charlie's parting blast is a set of educational objectives he expects his residents to achieve—or at least be given the opportunity to achieve —on each rotation. He has threatened to cancel his "purchase" of these rotations if the educational objectives are not met. The dean has to decide whether the money gets paid out. Charlie has become quite a chess player, for a gunfighter. ᣚ

Perhaps there were not enough gunfighters. Nationally, family practice had a difficult time establishing itself on an equal footing with other specialties. Internal medicine was too deeply entrenched, and internists had too much at stake to give up their turf (or give it back) to general practitioners, even if they were newly refurbished and packaged with a specialist label. This was especially true in academic medical centers. It was relatively easy to set up a family practice residency program in a community hospital, but not so easy in a university hospital.

Congress, disturbed by the profession's stalling on its 1971 initiative, passed even stronger legislation in 1976. The new Health Professions Educational Assistance Act (P.L. 94-484), however, pushed primary care, not just family practice. Apparently, the internists' and pediatricians' lobby got through, for both specialists were included in the definition of primary care. Congress was adamant about reversing the trend toward specialization. One clause in the law required a medical school to have 50% of its *first-year* residencies in primary care or lose its capitation grants for funding undergraduate medical education.

Yale and several other universities told the government, politely, to go to hell. They took umbrage at this attempt to interfere with the educational process and countered that they could do without the capitation grants. Other schools, however, less well endowed, changed their programs to conform to the letter of the law. Even so, Congress's big stick was really a rubber bat, easily pushed aside. Many students chose a flexible first year, the equivalent of the old internship, and then began to specialize in their second year. Actually, in internal medicine, specialization rarely begins until after the third year, in what are known as fellowships. The law simply failed to consider that students might switch to specialties later in the training period.

The 1976 law is a good example of how difficult it is to change the medical profession through legislation unless the profession agrees to the change. And Congress's hit-and-miss approach to health legislation—encouraging expansion one year and retrenchment the next—didn't help. There was no long-range plan, no national health policy, just a series of Band-Aids.

In 1976, however, the government also tried a new tactic in an attempt to solve the manpower problem. The Secretary of Health, Education, and Welfare (HEW)—now Health and Human Services (HHS)—established the Graduate Medical Education National Advisory Committee (GMENAC). This committee was to be a cooperative effort between government and the profession, a chance to work together. The committee was charged to "advise the Secretary on the number of physicians required in each specialty to bring supply and requirements into balance, methods to improve the geographic distribution of physicians, and mechanisms to finance graduate medical education."

At least they were trying.

CHAPTER 9

The Tragedy of the Medical Commons

IN THE EARLY 1970s, no one in government thought of controlling runaway costs by reestablishing the medical marketplace and allowing a laissez-faire free enterprise system to bring supply and demand into balance. There were many reasons for this. Medical care was still viewed as a sacred cow, not as an ordinary commodity suitable for trading in the marketplace. The liberals in Congress were still trying to enact some form of national health insurance legislation. And perhaps people thought that, like the government itself, the health care industry had grown so big, so out of hand, there was no hope of turning it back. But the simple fact is that *the law of supply and demand just doesn't work in medical practice.*

It is not that physicians don't believe in it; they just bypass it, as they would a blocked coronary artery. *Physicians supply their own demand.* Patients don't demand this laboratory test or that operation; physicians tell them what they need and then sell it to them.

Each physician has only one model to sell of whatever it is the patient has been told he or she can't live without. It's not like buying a car; you can't buy a low-, medium-, or high-priced model, any one of which will get you where you want to go. In medical care, you always get the high-priced model, whether you need all the accessories or not (some of these you purchase just to make sure the physician can't be charged with negligence). And, of course, the more you buy, the more the physician makes. That's why physicians want to hang on to fee-for-service reimbursement.

There is one economic law, however, that does apply to medicine. It's the law that states: If three stores on the same block are selling the same product, together they will do more than three times the business a single store alone would do on that block. One might expect that if two surgeons in partnership took in a third surgeon, the new surgeon would simply ease the workload of the other two. Not so. All three find more work to do. If you add three internists and a handful of other specialists—stand back, you might be trampled in the rush. Physicians stumbled onto this law when they started working in groups. It probably explains why they tend to congregate in one medical building and to move to suburbia, where the other doctors are.

It would be easy for government to control the health care industry if the usual economic laws applied. If it only had to identify the specific amount of medical care needed by a specific group of consumers, as the Graduate Medical Education National Advisory Committee was set up to do, then it would be easy to plan. It would know how many of each type of specialist and how many primary care physicians to order, how many nurses, how many technicians, how many hospitals, how many beds, how many X-ray machines, how many of this and that. But it doesn't work that way.

In medical practice, there has always been room for one more of anything. No matter how many doctors are added, even in overdoctored areas, there is always work for them. If you add ten more X-ray machines, they'll be used. If you add ten more beds, doctors will fill them. It may not be a law but it is an economic fact of life: If it's there, it will be used.

Government did try to take advantage of this economic fact of life to control costs when it enacted the National Health Planning and Resources Development Act in 1974 (P.L. 93-641). The idea was that if one controlled the capital investment in new facilities and technological equipment, this limitation of resources would slow utilization and curb the escalation of costs—if it wasn't there, it couldn't be used. The law required states to enact certificate-of-need legislation to implement this kind of control. But the bureaucratic red tape involved in setting up health service areas, administered by health system agencies, made for such a monster that the program ended up costing more than it saved. (It was one of the first programs earmarked for the scrap heap by the Reagan administration.)

Still, the concept was good, and it was used successfully by the private sector in regional health planning. In Philadelphia, for example, various business concerns got tired of being approached by every hospital in town for contributions to individual building campaigns. So in the 1960s they organized the Duane Committee to scrutinize the need for particular building programs and recommend which ones should be supported by the business community and which should not. This committee eventually became the local planning agency for the area under the Comprehensive Health Planning Act (P.L. 89-749) of 1966. And it is probably responsible for keeping health costs in Philadelphia much lower than those in the rest of the country, even today. Other business coalitions for health (of which there are now about sixty in major cities throughout the country) promise to assume a similar role in cost control (see Chapter 12).

Yet another strategy used by the government in its campaign to keep costs under control was regulation of the utilization of resources. The original Medicare and Medicaid legislation provided for review of the utilization of benefits. The fiscal intermediary was charged with monitoring utilization through its review of claims; it could deny payment for any care it judged unnecessary. The day-to-day review of utilization, however, was left to the medical staff of the hospital collectively and the admitting physician individually.

The physician was required to certify on the medical record that hospitalization of the patient was medically necessary. The medical staff committee had to monitor and approve the length of stay (LOS) for each admission and to verify the medical necessity of the specific services the physician provided. A hospital could not participate in the Medicare and Medicaid programs unless such a program of utilization review was in operation.

It might have looked good on paper, but the program was doomed from the start. Physicians saw the government as deputizing them—against their will—to be watchdogs for the federal dollars. More important, they resented that a clerk in an insurance company could overrule a physician's opinion. Retrospective denial of payment by the intermediaries was frequent, requiring long and complicated appeals if physicians disagreed (which they usually did).*

What the government failed to realize is that the physician alone determines when, where, and which medical resources need to be used. Only the physician is capable of determining the medical necessity of care; and the only utilization review program that can hope to succeed is one that has the full support and cooperation of the physicians involved— one they believe to be in the best interests of their patients.

Moreover, in attempting to regulate the use of resources, the government overlooked an important factor. Politicians kept calling for more doctors. What they failed to realize was that the more physicians, the more disease will be discovered. It isn't that doctors cause disease; usually they don't. (Although there is *iatrogenic*, or doctor-induced, disease and *nosocomial*, or hospital-acquired, illness; see Chapter 15.) But they certainly know where to find disease when it's least expected.

* This review system was replaced by the Professional Standards Review Organizations (PSRO) set up with the 1972 amendments to Medicare and Medicaid (P.L. 92–603). But this is a long story, and it is described more fully in Chapter 10.

It's like walking through a grove of oak trees; one would never know there were truffles buried around the roots of those trees. But walk through that grove with a pig or a pregnant poodle and look out—there will be an epidemic of truffles. Physicians were expert detectors of infected tonsils and diseased uteri, and, at least until recently, these organs were fair game. Ten years ago, if three children in the same family all had their tonsils out the same day, they would have their picture in the local newspaper. Today, their ENT (ear, nose, and throat) specialist would be reprimanded by the local peer review committee. And any hysterectomy performed on a woman under twenty-six would be suspect.

Yet even improved standards of care and active quality-control programs policed by physician peer review groups haven't totally changed the picture. The profession still believes that if you find something and there is something you can do about it, you do it. This is considered ethical practice. Physicians believe every patient comes to them with the request, usually not verbalized: "Do everything you can for me, Doc, no matter what it costs." To do otherwise would be unethical.

As our knowledge and technology have increased, as the physician can do more and more, medical practices have been introduced that may be beneficial to the individual but are not in the best interests of society. Dialysis for end-stage kidney disease is a case in point. These patients number less than 0.2% of Medicare beneficiaries, yet they utilize 5% of Medicare funds.

Other practices, now technically possible, benefit neither the individual nor society. For many diseases, one-third of the cost of all treatment is consumed in the last few days by keeping the patient alive on life-support systems, even though death is known to be inevitable. It takes a special court order in most hospitals to die peacefully; otherwise, the "deceased" will be subjected to attempts at cardiopulmonary resuscitation.

Physicians' urge to treat stems from a historical tradition: First, do no harm; but then do everything possible for the individual patient. Traditionally, cost has been of no concern—if patients couldn't pay, they couldn't pay; they were treated free. And physicians have always seen medical care resources as infinite. The little black bag had no bottom. Whatever was needed could be stuffed inside. And in today's world, with society providing the little black bag, that belief is all the stronger. As long as a treatment is known, it can be pulled out of the bag.

But this attitude is wrong. Our health care resources are finite. There is a bottom to the bag.

Certainly, many physicians would disagree with this statement. They believe our resources are not finite; it's simply a matter of national priorities. How can a nation that spends more on cosmetics each year than it does on education worry about the cost of health care?

Yet there must be some limit to the amount of its gross national product a country can spend on health care. What is the correct amount? Is it the 4.5% we were spending in 1950, the 9.8% we are spending now, 15%, 25%? One could suggest facetiously that if the increase continues at its present rate, by the middle of the twenty-first century we will be spending 100% of our GNP on health care—no army, no navy, no schools, no new highways; just more doctors, nurses, ambulances, and CAT scanners. Everyone will live happily ever after on life-support systems. Funeral homes will be out of date.

Ridiculous? Yes, But how far are we from the ridiculous? Are we not approaching the border?

Our per capita personal health care expenditures have increased from $70 in 1950 to over $1,200 in 1982. Yet some of the major items in this increase—the highly expensive new technology, new procedures, and new medications—have not been shown to have a clear cost benefit. It seems reasonable to require a demonstration of the correlation between the new technology and improved outcomes for treatment before we allocate more of our GNP to the Medical Establishment.

We, the consumers, pay the bill. We have a right to know that we are not just buying our doctors new toys to play with, toys that will be of no value in terms of our longevity or the quality of our life. There is a limit to the amount we can spend, especially if we do not know the value of what we are being asked to buy. We must tell the Medical Establishment that we do have finite resources.

In December 1968, an article called "The Tragedy of the Commons" appeared in *Science*, the journal of the American Association for the Advancement of Science. The author was Garrett Hardin, professor of biology at the University of California. Then, in July 1975, Howard Hiatt, dean of Harvard's School of Public Health, applied Hardin's "tragedy" to the field of medicine. His article, entitled "Protecting the Medical Commons: Who Is Responsible?", was published in the *New England Journal of Medicine*.

I first read these articles in the summer of 1977, while I was enrolled in the executive program in health services management at the Harvard Business School. I have reread them again and again, as one would a Bible. I believe them to be works of prophecy, enunciating specific concepts and considerations that must be followed if our contemporary health care system is to find its way to the promised land of optimal, affordable, quality health care for all our people.

In "The Tragedy of the Commons," Hardin discusses a class of contemporary problems characterized by a situation in which the resources are finite and insufficient to satisfy the total maximum demands that society might make. He likens this class of problems to the dilemma of a group of herdsmen whose cattle share a common pasture. As long as the number of animals is small in relation to the grazing capacity of the pasture, each herdsman can increase the size of his herd without detriment to the general welfare. As the number of cattle approaches the capacity of the land, however, each additional animal contributes to overgrazing. A single herdsman, attempting to maximize his own gain, can reasonably expect that the addition of one or just a few more cattle to his holdings will have minimal effect on the general welfare. All herdsmen, however, reasoning and acting individually in this manner, will destroy the commons. "Ruin," augurs Hardin, "is the destination toward which all men rush, each pursuing his own best interest in a society that believes in the freedom of the commons. Freedom in a commons brings ruin to all."

Hardin further believes that this kind of problem has no technical solution. He defines a technical solution as one that requires a change only in the techniques of the natural sciences, demanding little or nothing in the way of change in human values or ideas of morality. And he concludes, for example, that there is no technical solution to the world's problem of overpopulation; its solution will require a fundamental revision of our present-day morality.

Hiatt, in his article, calls on physicians individually and collectively to regard our health care resources as finite and to protect their use as one would protect a common pasture. "In our society," he explains, "demands from both preventive and curative medicine are made upon the same commons and, therefore, must be regarded as in competition with each other and with the needs for research and teaching."

Specifically, each physician goes to the commons for the resources he or she believes a patient should have, frequently using more than is essential for treatment. Any single physician could reasonably believe that one or two extra days in the hospital, a few more lab tests, or medications that aren't absolutely essential would have minimal effect on the general welfare. All doctors, however, reasoning and acting in this way, have managed to build the Medical Establishment to a size that far exceeds our needs. To meet the demands, we already have had to enlarge the commons, to allocate more of our GNP. Yet the demands are not always essential; precious resources are being used for practices that benefit neither the individual nor society.

New technologies are also raiding the commons. Few constraints are placed on the introduction of new medical practices. Many are introduced without adequate testing, without consideration of the long-term consequences. The Food and Drug Administration does require clinical trials before any new drug is put on the market, but there is no effective control over new instrumentation or new medical and surgical procedures. Certainly, no cost-benefit studies are done.

Clinical trials would provide the data necessary to make an informed decision on which of several vying options for health programs should be funded. As it stands now, Congress decides on program funding more or less arbitrarily, with no analysis of cost benefit. For example, no investigation was conducted before implementing the end-stage renal disease program (kidney dialysis), which initially required a $400 million annual allocation for a life extension benefit of four years for about 20,000 people (see Chapter 18). Might not that money have been better spent on a hypertension control program, which could have increased life expectancy by eighteen years for a much larger segment of our population?

"Willy-nilly coverage of special interest groups is a luxury we can no longer afford," contends Hiatt. "As we develop more and more practices that may be beneficial to the individual but not to the interest of society, we risk reaching a point where marginal gains to individuals threaten the welfare of the whole."

If we are to preserve the medical commons, all practitioners will eventually have to make cost-benefit judgments of alternative courses of action available in the medical armamentarium. Such decisions are especially crucial for conditions we have to treat with stopgap remedies because we do not know their real cause or their real cure. The choice among the various modalities for treating cancer is one example. On the other hand, when we do know the cause and can prevent a disease—by vaccinating for polio, for instance—we already know the cost benefit. There is no question of the many dollars that can be saved by preventing a disease. Given that few deaths have occurred with immunization programs, the cost seems small against the millions of lives that can be saved.

But to have physicians change the way they use the medical commons will not be easy. It would help if informed consumers demanded a change. Most physicians are waiting for a technical solution to the problems; as students of the Flexner era they are prone to do this and it is understandable. Most people prefer solutions that do not require them to relinquish rights and privileges they currently enjoy. Physicians are no different. They rationalize their position emotionally, based on accepted concepts of individual freedom and the belief in a laissez-faire enterprise system. They need to be told otherwise.

Hardin urges us to reexamine some of our concepts in the light of a changing world. We have not found solutions to many of our current problems, he claims, because Adam Smith's economic theory, which took hold in 1776, dominates our thinking. We still fundamentally believe that "decisions reached individually will, in fact, be the best decisions for an entire society; that an individual who intends his own gain is led by an invisible hand to promote the public interest." This belief, argues Hardin, leads to "the tragedy of the commons."

The only way to avoid the tragedy, according to Hardin, is to institute "mutual coercion, mutually agreed upon by the people affected." While we may not like this, because it diminishes our individual freedom, the alternatives may be even less to our liking.

Of course, individual physicians must continue to be free to provide all medically necessary care. At the same time, however, they must assure the continued freedom of medical practice by protecting the medical commons. They should avoid such practices as hospitalizing patients who can be treated equally well on an ambulatory basis. When hospitalization is required, they should manage and coordinate the care to avoid unnecessarily prolonged stays. They should not order laboratory studies automatically but choose only those that are really needed. They should use generic drugs when these are biologically equivalent or known to produce the same results. Instead of routine annual physical examinations, they should conduct periodic health assessments at intervals determined by the age, sex, and past history of the individual patient. They should take the time to develop a rapport with their patients so that they need not practice defensive medicine to protect themselves against malpractice. Overall, they should avoid any practices that benefit neither the patient nor society—some of which are discussed later in this book.

As Hardin says, individuals who misuse the commons "are free only to bring on universal ruin. Once they see the necessity of mutual coercion, they become free to pursue other goals. Freedom is the recognition of this necessity."

These words were written in 1968. Today, physicians are still waiting for a technical solution to the problem of the rising costs of medical care. None will come as long as they continue their blind love affair with technology, providing care that is not needed just because they are technically capable of providing it. The solution will require a change in physicians' thinking about their responsibilities in a free enterprise system of medical care. Forcing this change through the imposition of law or regulation will not work. It must come about by "mutual coercion, mutually agreed upon" by an enlightened medical profession.

CHAPTER 10

Mutual Coercion
Can Work

THERE IS one outstanding example of mutual coercion, instituted voluntarily by physicians to control utilization of hospital resources, that worked extremely well—until it became required by law. But first, some background information.

By conservative estimate, we have 25% more hospital beds than we need in the United States. Our hospitals are currently 75% occupied. For hospital administrators, the rule of thumb is that 85% occupancy is the most efficient and the most easy to manage; it's convenient for the medical staff and allows the patient population to find a bed when it's needed. When a hospital exceeds this 85% "norm," the administrator begins thinking about a building campaign to increase the bed capacity of the hospital. When the occupancy falls to 75% or lower, physicians are actively recruited to bring the occupancy back up to the norm. In the interim, the administrator explains away the empty "extra beds" as being necessary in an emergency. Yet it has been repeatedly observed that in an emergency, such as the recent nurses' strike in New York City, about 50% of hospitalized patients can be discharged immediately without risk to their welfare.

The practice of citing a high occupancy rate as a valid reason for requesting an increase in bed capacity—a common practice under certificate-of-need laws—has been shown to be completely invalid in a study by John Wennberg and Alan Gittelsohn published in the April 1982 *Scientific American*. In their article, entitled "Variations in Medical Care among Small Areas," they also indicate that the norm of 4 beds per 1,000 population—the standard under the Federal Health Planning Program (P.L. 93-641)—is not a satisfactory yardstick at the community level; it works only for large regions, such as a state.

Wennberg and Gittelsohn divide the six New England states into 193 hospital service areas based on data showing where the residents of surrounding communities (determined by zip code or township boundaries) actually go for hospital care. The number of beds in these service areas ranges from 6.8 per 1,000 to fewer than 2 per 1,000. Occupancy rates of hospitals in adjacent areas can vary considerably. The study suggests that the number of hospital beds depends more on the institution's priorities than on the needs of the population it services. In addition, the authors report:

Where there are many hospital beds per capita and many physicians whose specialty or style of practice requires frequent hospitalization, there is more treatment in hospitals and more expenditure per capita for hospital care. In hospital areas where there are many general surgeons the surgery rate is high. In areas where there are many internists many diagnostic tests are given. *The total rate of surgery and the likelihood of being admitted to a hospital for treatment thus depend on the supply of physicians and hospital beds in the area.* [Italics added.]

In one city in Maine the rate of hysterectomy (removal of the uterus) is so high that 75% of the women will have had the operation by the time they are seventy-five years old. Yet in an adjacent community, less than twenty miles away, the rate is much lower; only 25% of the women will have had the operation by the age of seventy-five. The rates of three of the most common surgical procedures (hysterectomy, prostatectomy, and tonsillectomy) vary sixfold from service area to service area. The study concludes that *"the amount and cost of hospital treatment in a community have more to do with the number of physicians there, their medical specialties and the procedures they prefer than with the health of residents."* (Italics added.)

The cost of hospital care in New England also varies with where one lives; it has nothing to do with one's health status. Medicare reimbursement to each person enrolled in the program in 1975 in Boston averaged $640. "Across the Charles River in Cambridge the amount was $540. In Manchester, New Hampshire, less than fifty miles away, it was $176." The amount spent per capita on hospital care also varied considerably in 1975, even in areas where the majority of admissions were to large teaching hospitals. In Boston, $324 per capita was spent; in Providence, $225; in New Haven, $153; and in Hanover, New Hampshire, $120.

The cost to the individual of hospital care in New England may not vary with where one lives. In some insurance programs it is obvious that those who live in New Hampshire are underwriting the higher cost of care in Boston. Take Medicare Part B (coverage of physicians' services), for example. Within the state of Vermont alone, it appears that residents in some areas are subsidizing the higher cost of hospital care in others. A study of sixteen service areas in Vermont in 1972 (when the premium for Part B supplemental coverage was $68 per individual, matched by another $68 by the government) showed that the per capita reimbursement for this coverage varied fourfold. In one area, the residents received services worth less than their $68 premium. In ten areas, residents received reimbursements of somewhere between $68 and $136 (the total premium for the coverage, including the government's contribution). In five areas, the residents benefited by payments in excess of $136 (in one area the reimbursement was $200 per capita).

Of course, the purpose of insurance is to spread the risk of medical care over a large number of people so no one individual has to pay the actual cost of needed care. But in this case, the risk seems to include the possibility not only of becoming ill but also of choosing a physician who is using the medical commons at a high rate.

There is no doubt that it is the physician who is responsible for the cost of hospital care. It is the physician who determines who is to be admitted to a hospital, which tests and treatments are ordered, which drugs are prescribed, and how long the patient stays. Within certain limits, it is also the physician's skill that determines whether or not there are complications in the course of treatment. Most hospital administrators will admit that the physician determines about 85% of hospital costs.

In Wennberg and Gittelsohn's study, information on the variation in the number of tonsillectomies performed was reported to the Vermont Medical Society. In the service area with the highest rate, physicians decided to require a second opinion before a tonsillectomy could be performed. The result was remarkable; the probability that a child would lose his or her tonsils before the age of twenty decreased from 60% to less than 10%. Residents of the area were closely monitored to see if they would go to neighboring areas to have their children's tonsils removed. They did not—"implying that demand by residents for the procedure had not been a major factor in maintaining the high tonsillectomy rate."

In discussing how the conditions identified in their study might be corrected, Wennberg and Gittelsohn point to the need for "an informed consumer of medical services."

When patients are aware that different forms of treatment are available, they can demand information on risks and benefits and make their own preferences known. If they know that rates of surgery are high at the local hospital, they may choose another. If they realize that a particular operation is a controversial one, they may seek the opinion of a second and even a third physician. Informed patients may, therefore, be the most important factor in making rates of treatment reflect health needs and eliminating unnecessary medicine.

Wishful thinking? Perhaps. It takes time for the consumer to become informed. Until the public gets around to taking physicians off the pedestal they have occupied for the past fifty years, it will be up to the profession to change the status quo. And physicians have changed things in some parts of America—which brings us back to our example of mutual coercion that worked.

In California, some physicians have been using half as many hospital beds as the rest of the country for the past twenty years. Moreover, they can document that the care their patients have received is of the highest quality.

The most accurate expression of hospital utilization is patient-days per 1,000 population. The current national rate of filling hospital beds is well over 1,000 patient-days per 1,000 (1,212, to be exact). (The 1980 data released by the AMA showed 159.5 admissions per 1,000 population for an average length of stay of 7.6 days; $159.5 \times 7.6 = 1,212$.) Yet, in California, county medical societies have formed "foundations for medical care" to conduct peer review of utilization, and they have kept hospital utilization for their members' patients under 500 patient-days per 1,000 for the past twenty years. One year, not long ago, the San Joaquin Foundation for Medical Care, the oldest of these organizations, recorded 329 patient-days per 1,000. So it can be done.

It all began in the mid-1950s. The San Joaquin County Medical Society was scared to death. It had just heard that the Kaiser-Permanente Plan was going to open an office in Stockton. The Kaiser Corporation had started the plan during World War II to provide medical care for employees and their families at plant sites far removed from existing medical services. The plan worked, and it was expanded after the war to several areas in California. It was also opened to the public. The Kaiser Plan offered total health care services to its enrollees for an annual premium of little more than what most health insurance plans were charging for coverage of in-hospital care alone. Kaiser included office visits and medications.

The Kaiser Plan combined an insurance company, a hospital, and a closed panel of physicians working in a group practice. (It later became the model for health maintenance organizations, discussed in the next chapter.) A single corporation ran the insurance company and the hospital facilities; this corporation (Kaiser Foundation Health Plan, Inc.) then contracted with the physician group (the Permanente Medical Group) to provide medical services. The contract with the medical group contained a financial incentive not to overutilize benefits. The group was paid an annual capitation fee for each enrollee to cover all his or her medical needs. At the end of the year, any unused portion of the capitation fee could be kept by the physician group. If use of benefits exceeded the capitation fee, the group was expected to provide this care free of charge.

This financial incentive worked; the Kaiser Plan experienced a 50% reduction in days of use of acute, short-term hospital care. Consequently, its lower premiums caused a serious economic challenge to the usual fee-for-service type of medical practice. Faced with such competition, it is no wonder the San Joaquin physicians were frightened.

But they didn't cower. Led by one of their members, Dr. Don Harrington, the doctors in San Joaquin County Medical Society met this challenge to their home turf head on. They set out to kill two birds with one stone; not only would they beat Kaiser at its own game, but they would show that fee-for-service solo practice, which most Americans preferred, was still better than group practice.

They approached insurance companies with the proposition that if the insurance benefits were expanded to cover office practice as well as hospital care, the physicians would form a voluntary organization, a foundation for medical care, separate from the county medical society, to control the use of benefits. All insurance claims by participating physicians would be reviewed by peers. Occidental Insurance Company was the first to take them up on their offer, and the doctors began the business of claims review.

This utilization control mechanism also worked. Other county medical societies followed San Joaquin's lead, and their foundations achieved the same 50% reduction in use of acute, short-term hospital care that Kaiser had. With retrospective denial of payment for claims that the peer review committee believed were not medically necessary, it took only a short time for physicians to learn how to use the medical commons appropriately. Their peers were watching. Mutual coercion worked.

Meanwhile, back in Washington, Congress was writing the 1970 amendments to the Medicare and Medicaid programs. These programs had been in operation only four years, and already they had far exceeded their estimated budgets. Senator Wallace Bennett (R.–Utah) of the Senate Finance Committee was looking for a mechanism to control these costs.

The original law had mandated that the medical staff of a hospital had to have a utilization review program in order for the hospital to be paid for its Medicare and Medicaid patients. This committee of physicians was to review the appropriateness of admission and the length of stay for every patient. In practice, this review was often second-guessed by the claims-paying intermediary—by an insurance company, which made the final decision for Medicare patients, or by a state agency, which decided for Medicaid patients. Retrospective denial of payment was frequent, and the hospitals, the doctors, and the patients became extremely upset with the program. The reason this utilization review program didn't work was that physicians resented being forced against their will to police the government's health care dollar. Why should they bother, they thought, if the insurance intermediaries could overrule their opinion? A new means of cost control had to be found.

Senator Bennett decided to change this and give physicians the final say. If local practicing physicians could control hospital utilization in California, why not mandate this prototype throughout the country? The San Joaquin Foundation for Medical Care became the model.

The new physician organizations would be called Professional Standards Review Organizations (PSROs). They were to conduct concurrent reviews; that is, they were to determine the medical necessity of care, the appropriateness of hospitalization, and the required length of stay *while* the patient was still in the hospital. This *concurrent* review would remove the stigma of retrospective denial of payment. The insurance companies would continue to serve as the government's intermediaries in claims payment; but they would have to accept the PSROs' judgment on the medical necessity and appropriateness of hospital utilization.

I joined the staff of the American Hospital Association (AHA) as associate director in September 1970. This was one month after Senator Bennett had introduced his amendment. My first day on the job, Dr. Edwin Crosby, director of AHA and my immediate boss, assigned me to watch over this piece of legislation. "If you don't think hospitals can live with it, then figure out how to change it or how we can kill it," he said.

Hospitals could never have lived with the initial draft of this legislation. It was designed to control costs with no concern for quality. It became obvious to me that quality of care could deteriorate if only costs were being monitored. Cost and quality had to be reviewed simultaneously. The only way to do this would be to develop a cookbook approach to care. (Did you do this and that? Did you order this lab test? Do that X ray?) Such an approach would be totally unacceptable to physicians. The utilization review had to be coordinated with a medical audit, an existing technique that was used to measure quality of care and that was acceptable to most physicians.

The initial draft of the legislation also took the control mechanism out of the hospital and put it in the hands of physicians external to the institution—but only for Medicare and Medicaid patients. A potential result was a two-class system of health care, one for the poor and elderly and another for the rest of society. Moreover, this system would duplicate control mechanisms already in operation. Hospital law and the Joint Commission on Accreditation of Hospitals mandated that the medical staff of a hospital be responsible to the hospital governing authority for this utilization review for all patients.

Presented with these ideas, Senator Bennett modified his amendment to require PSROs to accept the findings of and delegate the authority to a hospital medical staff committee that was performing the function well to carry out the PSROs review within its institution, reporting to the PSROs and operating under guidelines set by the PSROs. The amendment, however, was not passed until 1972, when it became part of P.L. 92-603.

The delay gave the AHA an opportunity to develop a new program, called Quality Assurance, to make sure medical staff committees in hospitals functioned well. The Quality Assurance Program combined utilization reviews and medical audits so that cost and quality could be evaluated together and also meet all PSROs requirements. In a Quality Assurance Program, criteria are developed by the medical staff as standards to judge the quality of care provided for the individual patient. These criteria include appropriate tests to be done, complications to be avoided, and also proper utilization of resources, *i.e.*, length of stay and cost of care. Adequate care is measured against these standards, and deviation from quality is analyzed on a case-by-case basis.

Over 200 PSROs are in operation today throughout the United States, but no one knows whether or not they are effective. Certainly, they have not controlled the cost of hospital care, which has continued to rise annually at a higher rate than the Consumer Price Index. But then, what would the cost be if PSROs were not in place? No one has come up with a satisfactory evaluation. Dr. Helen Smits, who was responsible for the PSROs program during the Carter administration, admitted in a July 1981 article in the *New England Journal of Medicine* that it is impossible to provide the kind of evaluation the multiple layers of bureaucratic overseers demand. The Department of Health and Human Services, the Office of Management and Budget, the White House, and Congress all want a yes or no: Is it saving more than it is costing? Since no one can answer that question, the program will probably be given the axe by the Reagan administration.

My own evaluation is that the PSRO program has and hasn't worked. It depends on what one expects. It certainly has not worked as well as Senator Bennett predicted it would; it hasn't accomplished what the San

Joaquin Foundation for Medical Care continues to accomplish in terms of patient-days per 1,000 population. In 1968, we were utilizing 1,164 patient-days per 1,000; in 1980, that figure had risen to 1,212.

Looked at only in terms of length of stay, utilization review has been a success. We have chopped nearly a full day off each hospitalization—a decrease of almost 10%. Using the 1980 figures, at $245.12 per day times 0.8 days times 36.1 million admissions, we saved over $7 billion in 1980. The shorter length of stay has also decreased hospital occupancy by 6% since 1968, while use of outpatient services has increased 77%. In other words, we are utilizing hospitals much more efficiently. Productivity in the hospital field is measured in terms of how fast a bed can be turned over. On this basis, we are more productive. We have turned over our beds faster than in 1968, treated more people on an ambulatory basis, and seemingly saved a lot of money.

The problem is we are now admitting 9 million more patients per year than we were in 1968. It is not just that there are more people, although our population has grown. We are admitting 21 per 1,000 more than in 1968. It is these 9 million more admissions that have raised our total hospital bill. Were all these admissions medically necessary? The medical staff committees said they were, and the PSROs certified them as necessary. What's wrong, then, with the doctors in San Joaquin? Why don't they find 700 more patient-days per 1,000 medically necessary? Why aren't they like other doctors in keeping beds filled?

There is no doubt that coercion works only when it is mutually agreed upon by those being coerced. But why did the San Joaquin physicians agree to mutual coercion? Did they really understand the need to protect the medical commons? Or was it the competition from Kaiser that motivated them?

The government think tanks believe it was the competition. So a new government strategy is upon us. The theory is that if competition is created in the health field between different types of delivery systems, then there will be no need for government regulation. The free enterprise system will come into its own. The efficient, high-quality, low-cost system will survive and the inefficient, low-quality, high-cost system will go under.

The government thinks the new health maintenance organization is the efficient, high-quality, low-cost system and the traditional solo practice, fee-for-service system is the other. But let's examine this HMO concept and see if we want to live with it before we completely restructure our delivery system.

CHAPTER 11

Do Health Maintenance Organizations Really Maintain Health?

HEALTH MAINTENANCE ORGANIZATIONS (HMOs) became legitimate—at least they received their official name—on February 5, 1970, in the hotel suite of Dr. Paul Ellwood at the DuPont Plaza in Washington, D.C. Ellwood and his Minneapolis think tank were serving as consultants to the Nixon administration, which was looking for a Republican answer to halt the rising costs of Medicare and Medicaid.

Ellwood pointed out to Nixon's top brass in the health arena that our system for organizing and financing health care contained incentives that inflated costs. Basically, the system encouraged the overuse of highly specialized, technologically intensive institutional care. Medicare and Medicaid reimbursed this hospital care on a cost basis; that is, the higher the hospital's costs, the more it was paid.

The benefits were mainly designed to cover in-hospital care; there were only minimal ambulatory and preventive benefits. Doctors were paid on a fee-for-service basis, which meant that the more care they ordered, the more they were paid.

Ellwood believed that a reorganization of the delivery system and a change in the financing mechanism was needed in order to provide incentives for more efficient, cost-conscious care. He felt that if the incentives were changed, the system would respond.

He cited several examples of alternative delivery systems that had been operating successfully for many years with lower costs—including prepaid group practices, independent practice associations, and health care corporations. In all these organizations, a number of physicians were organized in some manner to provide comprehensive health care services for a specific time period, for a defined group of individuals, for a specified and predetermined price. Ellwood called these various models health maintenance organizations, the idea being that an HMO would have an incentive to maintain the health of its patients and reduce the incidence of disease.

Unfortunately, this is not exactly what has happened. Most HMOs limit health maintenance services to periodic health evaluations, with physical exams, routine immunizations, well-baby care, prenatal care, and minimal patient education. None that I have seen includes positive programs promoting health and wellness (discussed in detail in the second part of this book). Even in the largest and most successful HMO (Kaiser/Oakland), only 14% of the enrollees have been taking advantage of the limited health maintenance services to which they are entitled. The same is true for most HMOs because physicians must order health maintenance services for their patients, just as they need to order any service. And, as in the fee-for-service system, physicians are not doing this.

HMOs, however, do show a reduced use and, therefore, a reduced cost in hospital care. This is primarily owing to two factors. First, the financing mechanism, the capitation method of reimbursement, has removed the financial incentive for a physician to overutilize services. Second, HMOs generally enroll young, healthy, employed individuals, whose use of hospital care is less than that of the general public. HMOs have not generally been burdened with the high users—the disabled and the elderly.

HMO cost savings have not been accomplished by maintaining the health of the individual patient. This fact seems to be ignored by politicians who are advancing HMOs as the panacea for all of America's health care ills. They appear to really believe that these organizations are not only maintaining the health of their enrollees but also promoting health. Nothing could be further from the truth. The "health maintenance" name is pure Madison Avenue, good PR imaging, like the New York ice cream that is cleverly packaged to appear to have been made in Denmark.

Any HMO cost savings have been effected by the two factors previously mentioned: the capitation method of reimbursement and the selection of healthy enrollees. Still, the capitation method of reimbursement does hold advantages over existing fee-for-service and cost reimbursement methods. In the capitation method, a group of physicians is given a set fee each year by each individual who enrolls in the program, with the understanding that the group will provide all the individual's needs for medical care during that year. The physicians are thereby placed at risk in providing care for their enrollees. If the money runs out before the end of the year, they can't go back to the enrollees and ask for more. On the other hand, if the physicians work efficiently, there may be money left over at the end of the year, and they can keep this as a bonus. Obviously, it's to the physicians' advantage not to overutilize resources by ordering unnecessary tests or putting a patient into the hospital when ambulatory treatment would be just as effective. (There is also an incentive to keep enrollees healthy—but, unfortunately, physicians have yet to explore this advantage.)

All health and medical care needs must come out of the capitation fee, including hospital care, which receives the largest share of the capitation dollar. Some physician groups, such as the Independent Practice Association, and other HMOs purchase hospital care from several hospitals, but most prepaid group practice models of HMOs usually own their hospital. It is perhaps easiest to understand the group practice model of the HMO, of which the Kaiser Plan is the best example.

As we have already seen, Kaiser Foundation Health Plan has three components: a corporate insurance and administrative arm; Kaiser Foundation hospitals, which the corporation owns and operates; and the Permanente Medical Groups, a professional association of physicians organized in a group practice, which contracts with the corporation to provide all medical care for enrollees of the plan. Whether you call it an HMO or a prepaid group practice, the Kaiser Plan provides very realistic incentives to contain health care costs. Compared with the fee-for-service or cost reimbursement system, this capitation system requires one-fourth to one-third fewer hospital beds to care for enrollees. Available beds are turned over faster and fewer patients are admitted. The average length of stay in the Kaiser hospitals is usually under five days, compared with about seven and a half days nationwide. This is increased productivity as we previously defined it—faster turnover of fewer beds.

Kaiser physicians admit fewer patients to the hospital because they treat more on an ambulatory basis. It is claimed that because access to primary care is easier in an HMO, problems are diagnosed earlier, before the patients reach a degree of illness that requires hospitalization. Kaiser also uses many more primary-care physicians than specialists; the ratio is 2:1. Whatever the reason, Kaiser has kept its rate of hospital utilization to less than 500 patient-days per 1,000 enrollees, compared with our national average of 1,212 patient-days per 1,000 people.

This saving in high-cost hospital care can be used to cover more ambulatory care in the physicians' offices. In other words, the HMO can provide comprehensive care, with ambulatory as well as hospital benefits, for the same premium that Blue Cross/Blue Shield and indemnity health insurance companies charge for in-hospital benefits only.

Despite the proven cost containment advantages of HMOs, neither health care providers nor the American public has enthusiastically embraced them. Hospitals see no advantage in contracting with an HMO as long as cost reimbursement prevails. Why should they place themselves at risk if they don't have to? But should cost reimbursement be discontinued and replaced by prospective rate setting, a hospital administrator might be sorely tempted to contract with an HMO, which can guarantee 10,000 admissions to the hospital per year, rather than continue to deal with the vagaries of 150 individual medical staff members.

Physicians' feelings are more intense. Why should they move to capitation reimbursement as long as fee-for-service payment is available? Like the hospitals, why should they place themselves at risk? Moreover, HMOs require a restructuring of the delivery system in which they might lose their freedom of individual action—a way of life that made many of them choose a career in medicine in the first place. Even an independent practice association, a lesser evil in their eyes than a prepaid group practice, infringes on their individual liberty. They prefer the status quo.

Organized medicine, the American Medical Association, has encouraged this thinking. It is glad now that it lobbied to have state legislatures enact laws forbidding the corporate practice of medicine. Although only twenty-two states passed such legislation, it has proved an effective barrier to the initiation of HMOs in those states.

Such prejudices die slowly. It is unlikely that the profession will be easily moved into approving HMOs. Besides, there is no groundswell from the American people pushing in this direction.

Most middle- and upper-income Americans have always believed that one of the most important elements in our present system of medical care is the patient's free choice of a physician. To be assigned a physician, or to be locked in with a particular physician for the rest of the year after a misunderstanding has arisen, is unacceptable to most. They prefer to have a family doctor of their own choosing and the free choice of a specialist when and if they need one. This insistence on freedom of choice is the one factor that will preserve our present delivery system despite its cost. Cost seems of secondary importance to most people when their health is at stake.

Free choice of a physician was a hallmark of the Medicare and Medicaid legislation enacted in 1965. It could not have passed unless it guaranteed this right. Many of the elderly refused to sign up for coverage until they were assured that their individual dignity would not be imposed upon.

The law also prohibited any reorganization of the delivery system. Medicaid, the health care financing program for the poor, reflected the social revolution of the 1960s, which demanded access to health care services as a right. The poor were not interested in having their care paid for in charity clinics—that had been their lot for too long. They wanted to be able to choose their own physicians and to see a physician in his or her office; again, it was an issue of human dignity.

Physicians who have worked in charity clinics also find this form of practice unacceptable, and my own experience bears this out. Clinic patients are simply assigned to whichever physician is available. Almost half the time spent with a patient must be used to determine what has gone before. Many times the records of previous physicians are incomplete. And it is nearly impossible to communicate to the next physician the nuances of the encounter—nuances that can be quite significant in the practice of good medicine.

Patients, too, become frustrated by having to repeat their medical history to every new physician they see. It destroys confidence in the system and prevents the close rapport and security of a good patient-physician relationship. Having to deal with a different physician each time can inhibit the patient's free exchange of information, so necessary for a physician to be able to give the best care.

Patients and physicians alike feel that it would be retrogressive to move from our present one-to-one relationship in the fee-for-service system to a group practice model (the predominant form of HMOs), where care of one patient is divided among several physicians. Many fear that the impersonal relationships characteristic of the old charity clinics will be repeated in HMOs, especially if HMOs are mandated in the federal Medicare and Medicaid programs. It was startling and frightening to hear Richard Schweiker, the recent Secretary of Health and Human Services, a Republican, advocating the elimination of free choice of physician in the Medicaid program.

Government, however, has had a different view of HMOs from that held by the providers and the public. Republicans and Democrats in government alike, from the Nixon administration through the Carter one, have seen HMOs as the means of changing the financing mechanism of health care and providing incentives to contain costs. Even Senator Edward Kennedy, when he realized the enactment of national health insurance legislation was unlikely, embraced HMOs. Kennedy sees them, however, as a first step toward national health insurance—a foot in the door. This view is shared by the AMA, although it evokes a totally different emotional response.

For all its support, Congress, in enacting legislation to promote HMOs, may have succeeded in killing them. Had this been its motive, it could not have written a better law. The legislation required that employers grant their employees a choice of an HMO as an alternative to the usual health insurance benefit if a federally qualified HMO existed in the community. To be federally qualified, an HMO had to provide specific benefits prescribed in the law. This benefit package, however, was so large and expensive that it priced HMOs out of competition with other health insurance programs.

The law also required that if there was any money left at the end of the year in the capitation pot, these savings had to be shared with the federal government. In one stroke, the government completely eliminated the financial incentives that had made HMOs successful in the private sector. It emasculated the HMO concept.

HMOs are difficult to start up even under the best of circumstances. An HMO must have a large enough number of enrollees to ensure that the total capitation fees for a year will cover the minimum expenses of the group. It usaully takes several years before an HMO can become financially viable on its own. Even Kaiser, with all its resources and experience, expects to subsidize a new branch operation for a minimum of two years.

The HMO legislation was designed to help subsidize the start-up phase through grants and loans until a new HMO had sufficient numbers of enrollees to survive. Initially, 75% of federally funded HMOs failed to survive because of the high cost-benefits package. The law was then amended to reduce the number of required benefits. Nevertheless, since then, only 50% have made it to the point of being self-sufficient or financially viable.

Despite all the failures, the government still has faith in the HMO. The Reagan administration sees the HMO as a key factor in its new strategy—competition. Is that what we need?

CHAPTER 12

Competition: The Government's New Strategy

THE 1970s will be remembered in health care history as a decade of frustration, ten years during which government tried without success to control health care costs. During the 1960s, government encouraged expansion of the Medical Establishment. During the 1970s, it turned to regulation, with the hope of slowing the growth it had fostered. The same problems remained; they just grew more intense.

Paul Ellwood put his finger on the problem in 1970 when he pointed out that our system contains perverse incentives that inflate costs (see Chapter 11). He felt that if the incentives were changed, the system would respond. He could be giving the same advice today; it is still pertinent.

Despite ten years of government regulation, nothing basic to the organization and financing of our delivery system has changed since 1970. We do have a few more health maintenance organizations, but the skeletons of the 50% that died before they reached maturity are strewn along the wayside. The survivors number just over 200, serving 5% of our population, with about 10 million enrollees. For the remaining 95% of our people, however, the basic system has not changed. It has just become more expensive.

Most of our insurance programs, including Medicare and Medicaid, still reimburse hospitals on a cost basis; the higher the costs a hospital incurs, the more it is paid. In the federal programs providing medical care for the poor and elderly, the effect is an open-ended redistribution of wealth that will become an increasing tax burden until the reimbursement method is changed.

In 1970, national health expenditures were $74.7 billion—7.6% of the gross national product. In 1980, they were $247.2 billion—9.4% of the GNP. One year later, in 1981, they had risen to $287 billion—9.8% of the GNP. What these figures mean is that in the past decade consumers have had to double the amount of real income (adjusted for inflation) they spend on medical care each year. Of course, the fact that people spend a larger percentage of their income on medical care—and relatively less on food, housing, education, vacations, and savings—is of little concern to the federal government. Nor should it be, *if* consumers want to spend their money on medical care. The problem is that they don't want to; they have no choice.

The government's concern is the rising expense of Medicare and Medicaid, which now cost $60 billion per year. If the government ends up having to bail out these programs with funds from general revenues, it won't be able to spend as much on defense, energy, transportation, or any of the other demands on federal revenues. Add to this the Reagan administration's insistence on balancing the budget to stem inflation, while simultaneously cutting taxes to stimulate the economy, and the cost of health care becomes a federal headache.

But the headache won't go away; it just seems to get worse. None of the remedies the government has tried has worked. The HMO strategy didn't relieve the pain. Nor did the other "medications," the attempts at regulation through price control, Professional Standards Review Organizations, health planning of capital investment, and certificate-of-need legislation. Ceilings on hospital costs were threatened by the Carter administration but were never passed by Congress. It's true the threat itself did prod providers to try to contain the rate of increase in what was called the Voluntary Effort. But once the threat of imposed ceilings was removed, the rate of increase in costs rose to where it was before. By this time, everyone was discouraged by the failure of regulation and was looking around for a new approach.

When Carter took office in 1976, he inherited a Medicare outlay of about $17.8 billion, with a projected 25% increase per year. Something had to be done. Joseph Califano, Secretary of Health, Education, and Welfare, sought outside consultation, and he turned to Alain C. Enthoven, an economist at Stanford's Graduate School of Business.

Enthoven told the Carter administration much the same as Ellwood had told the Nixon brass. But he went a few steps further. The basic system had the wrong incentives, he claimed, but government policies and programs were making it worse. Medicare, Medicaid, and the tax laws were not just subsidizing a profligate system; in effect, they were pouring gasoline on the fire of inflation. (My analogy, not his.)

Enthoven's report to Califano was published as a two-part article in the *New England Journal of Medicine* in the spring of 1978.* I quote:

The main cause of the unjustified and unnecessary increase in costs is the complex of perverse incentives inherent in the tax-supported system of fee for

---

* Alain C. Enthoven, "Consumer Choice Health Plan."

service for doctors, cost reimbursement for hospitals, and third-party intermediaries to protect consumers. Fee for service rewards the doctor for providing more and more costly services, whether or not more is necessary or beneficial to the patient. Cost reimbursement rewards the hospital with more revenue for generating more costs. . . . Third-party reimbursement leaves the consumer with, at most, a weak financial incentive to question the need for or value of services or to seek out a less costly provider or style of care.

The economic factors are important, but the important factors are not all economic. The financial incentives are reinforced by the demands and expectations of anxious patients, the prestige associated with costly technologic care, the malpractice-induced need for "defensive medicine," and the government-inspired proliferation of health manpower—especially physicians. Thus, the financing system rewards cost-increasing behavior and provides no incentive for economy.

Medical costs are straining public finances. Direct economic regulation will raise costs, retard beneficial innovation, and be increasingly burdensome to physicians. As an alternative, I suggest that the government change financial incentives by creating a system of competing health plans in which physicians and consumers can benefit from using resources wisely.

In such a system, costs can be controlled with freedom of choice that respects each person's preferences. But the distinctive idea of this proposal is to let consumer preferences guide the reorganization of the health care delivery system. I have called it Consumer Choice Health Plan (CCHP).

In his proposal, Enthoven envisioned physicians taking the responsibility to create organizations, such as HMOs or independent practice associations, capable of providing comprehensive health care services to defined populations of enrollees, financed by prospective per capita payment. They would compete in a free marketplace. The consumer would have the choice of which organization to use. The cost and quality of benefits provided would govern the consumer's choice of organization, forcing the delivery system to reorganize itself to conform to the needs of the consumer. Enthoven believed that physicians would be forced by economic means to change from fee-for-service to capitation reimbursement and hospitals from cost reimbursement to prospective rates, in order to compete.

Government, he said, should not force the system upon us—the public would reject such involuntarily imposed changes—but rather stimulate its genesis by providing tax incentives for those who chose this type of delivery system. The present system should be permitted to remain intact until economic pressures of competition force it to change voluntarily.

For Enthoven's consumer choice strategy to work, an important element in our current system—third-party reimbursement—needs to be changed. At present, most consumers do not deal directly with the provider in paying for medical care; an intermediary—the third party—handles the bill.

It's like going shopping in Saks Fifth Avenue with your doctor and a magic credit card. Your doctor tells you to buy this and that, one of these and two of those. "You really need this, Mabel," the expert says, "it'll do wonders for you." So you buy it and give the clerk your card. You don't care how much the items cost because you have this magic credit card.

This card is nothing like your American Express or Visa card, where you have to pay up at the end of the month. With your magic credit card you have to pay only a set amount each month no matter how much you buy. Of course, you pay the same amount each month whether you use it or not, but when you do go shopping for medical care it's magic! You can buy as much as you want as long as your doctor says it's okay and you don't have to worry about the cost of anything. Of course, after you have spent a certain amount you may find that the card covers only 80% of the cost. But it's still a great bargain even if some cards make you pay cash for the first thing you buy each year; after that the sky's the limit. No question, it's magic.

Enthoven says that if we didn't have magic credit cards we would be more prudent buyers. We would have to go shopping with only cash in our pockets. If our doctor said to buy this, we would probably ask the price first. If we felt we couldn't afford it, we might ask our doctor if we really needed it. Or we might try the basement sales, to see if we could get just as good quality for a lower price. Enthoven's ideas caught the imagination of Democrats and Republicans alike. Perhaps, at last, the present system could be turned around and headed in the right direction. Especially appealing was the fact that many of Enthoven's ideas could be instituted piecemeal—without calling it national health insurance. Enthoven himself suggested that "incremental changes should be made in the present system to alter it fundamentally, but gradually and voluntarily. Freedom of choice for consumers and physicians should be preserved."

All the bright young politicians saw the potential in Enthoven's ideas. In 1979, Representative Richard Gephardt (D.–Mo.) and Representative David Stockman (R.–Mich.) cosponsored a consumer choice competition bill in the House. In the Senate, Richard Schweiker (R.–Pa.) and David Durenberger (R.–Minn.) each sponsored bills. *Consumer choice* became the new buzzword in Washington.

With the change in administrations and the start of the 97th Congress, the concept grew. But the buzzword changed to *competition*, a much more Republican term.

Two sponsors of consumer choice competition bills in the 96th Congress were given important posts in the Reagan administration. David Stockman became the new director of the Office of Management and Budget. Richard Schweiker became the new Secretary of Health and Human Services. Schweiker quickly appointed two task forces to draft a competition strategy for the administration.

Representative Gephardt reintroduced his bill in the new Congress as H.R. 850. Senator Orrin Hatch (R.–Utah) sponsored the same bill that Schweiker had introduced in the previous Congress (S. 139), and Senator Durenberger reintroduced his bill (S. 433). Note that Gephardt is a member of the House Ways and Means Committee; Hatch is Chairman of the Senate Labor and Human Resources Committee; and Senator Durenberger is Chairman of the Senate Finance Subcommittee on Health. All these committees deal with health legislation. Thus, the competition advocates are in a good position to encourage passage of a competition bill, especially if one is pushed by the White House.

These various bills are similar in concept and are based on Enthoven's basic idea. They deal with the mechanism for government to provide the financial incentives for the new system. Most plans are designed to recast the government subsidy Americans now enjoy in the form of a tax deduction to cover our health insurance premiums.

The major subsidy comes through our employers. The health insurance premium provided by our employers is tax deductible for them and benefits are not taxable as income for us.

This government subsidy, however, is not applied equitably. Some employers provide greater benefits than others in the package of health insurance they buy. Some pay 100% of costs, not the usual 80% that requires a co-payment. Some give coverage from the first dollar; with others, the employee has to pay a deductible. Some include major medical for catastrophic illness, others do not.

We can look at this government subsidy as a form of national health insurance for the employed, paid out of otherwise taxable revenues. And we also have a kind of national health insurance for the elderly and disabled through Medicare, the poor through Medicaid, and for the Indians, Aleuts, Eskimos, military and their dependents, veterans and merchant marines through government medical services. The people who are not covered are the self-employed, the unemployed, and the near-poor. The near-poor are those who are employed only part time or are employed in such unskilled jobs that their employers do not provide health insurance; yet, their income is over the poverty level so they do not qualify for Medicaid. They form the largest group of the medically indigent. There are others, too, who are not covered by any federal program: the poor in Arizona, which until recently did not have a Medicaid program; the poor in states like Massachusetts, which has been unable to pay for the care of its Medicaid population and has turned much of the burden over to local governments; the elderly who do not have Social Security and do not qualify for Medicaid; and illegal aliens, who receive a large portion of the charity care provided by inner-city hospitals.

In all, there are probably 40 million to 50 million Americans who do not have some form of health insurance. But the government is already, directly or indirectly, subsidizing health care for the rest of the population. How can we change the inequities in this system? And how can we all become more prudent buyers?

Most proposals remove the tax exemption on the amount we receive from our employer in health benefits; it would then be taxable as income. To offset the tax on this increased income, however, we would be given a tax credit for a portion of the amount our employer contributed for health benefits if we used this credit to pay for health care from among the choices we were offered. Employers, on the other hand, would be allowed to claim employee health benefits as a business expense, up to a ceiling, as long as they offered a choice among several competing plans that were federally qualified.

To be federally qualified, a plan would have to provide minimum benefits and include catastrophe coverage. To prevent a plan from skimming (selecting only enrollees with a low health risk), all plans would be required to hold annual open enrollment and to charge all enrollees the same premium for the same benefits. The premiums, therefore, would be *community-rated* rather than experience-rated; that is, they would not be based on the individual's health status or history of previous use.

We, the employees, the consumers of health services, could choose among a range of plans, from one providing only basic benefits at low cost to one giving comprehensive coverage at high cost. We could also select a high-cost plan with no deductibles and no co-payment, or a low-cost one with considerable co-payment and deductibles. If we chose one that cost less than the amount of our employer's contribution, we would get a cash refund from the government for the difference. If we chose a more expensive plan, we would have to pay the difference out of our own pockets—which might make us think about costs.

The consumer choice plan is based on the Federal Employees Health Benefits Program (FEHBP), which has been operating successfully since 1959. It now covers 10.5 million federal employees. The government, as an employer, pays 60% of the average premium; the employee pays the rest. There are seventy-nine competing plans, including Aetna, BlueCross/ Blue Shield, and alternative delivery systems such as HMOs.

The competition strategy also envisions that Medicare and Medicaid will be replaced by a voucher system, in which the federal government assumes the role of the employer and pays the premium for the beneficiaries of these programs. The voucher can be used by the beneficiary to purchase one of several competing health plans.

The theory is that, if given a choice among competing health care plans, the consumer will choose the one offering the greatest benefits at the least cost. This will trigger a chain reaction that will change the system.

The providers of health care, the physicians and hospitals, will have an incentive to reorganize in various ways in order to compete for the consumer's dollar. It is anticipated that HMOs, including both prepaid group practice and independent practice associations, will have a financial advantage over fee-for-service solo practice, thereby forcing most physicians into one of these alternative forms of practice. (Studies have shown that total costs—premiums plus out-of-pocket costs—in an HMO are 10% to 40% lower than total costs in a fee-for-service system.)

These forces will restructure our delivery system by incremental evolution, claims Enthoven, rather than by direct government intervention. (Thus, government will be able to avoid the great anathema and follow the rule of "do no *direct* harm.")

Will it work? Can it work? Is it possible to turn around this behemoth, the Medical Establishment, with such a simple strategy? Many say yes and many say no. The consensus at this point in the debate is that it would take a major push by the President himself to overcome the opposition of many important lobbys.

The American Medical Association has gone on record as favoring many of the tenets of competition. But it is vehemently opposed to one aspect of the Gephardt-Stockman bill; it objects to any federal tampering with state laws that now restrict the corporate practice of medicine.

Industry appears to be opposed to the strategy, if one can gauge by the reaction of one of its most vocal constituents, the Washington Business Group on Health, composed of about 200 of the Fortune 500. Many employers have moved to self-insurance of their health care benefits, which gives them a handle on controlling costs. Competition would eliminate self-insurance; in 1981, 36% of the Fortune 500 companies were self-insured.

Labor is strongly opposed because it sees many of the hard-earned benefits it has gained through collective bargaining being wiped out. Industry agrees; health benefits have been an important bargaining tool.

The health insurance industry doubts that the strategy will work. Free choice of a lower cost may not be a strong enough incentive to change the status quo. It cites the fact that 65% of consumers in the FEHB program choose the high-benefits option with first-dollar coverage. The insurance industry's main fear is adverse selection, in which the young and healthy select the low-cost, low-benefit plans, leaving the high-cost comprehensive plans with the high-risk high-users. As a result, the base for sharing the risk of comprehensive plans would be limited and could price them out of competition.

The hospital field is divided on the issue. Cost reimbursement, which has been such a windfall to hospitals for the past fifty years, would be eliminated. But they would be relieved of much of the repressive regulation of the past ten years. The for-profit hospital groups are promoting the idea because they see it as a much more viable alternative than utility-type regulation, which could severely restrict their freedom of action.

The medical schools and teaching hospitals are adamantly against the strategy. Eighty percent of graduate medical education and clinical research is funded from patient revenues. They do not see how they could possibly compete on the basis of costs with community hospitals, which have only patient care responsibilities and thus much lower costs. Under competition, a new method of payment for graduate medical education would have to be found.

Consumers have generally not yet become involved in the debate. One opinion has come from lobbyists representing the elderly. They have voiced concern that some Medicare benefits may be lost and the elderly will be required to pay out more in deductibles and co-payment—money that many do not have. Many old people might then be forced to turn to Medicaid for help with a loss of dignity and independence. But wouldn't the same situation arise if nothing were done and costs kept escalating? Lobbyists have also questioned whether consumers will be able to judge alternative plans wisely. If they can't, the concept would seem unworkable.

And so the debate is heating up. The skeptics see the entire competition strategy as a smoke screen, thrown up for one purpose only—to permit the federal government to pass the costs of Medicare and Medicaid on to the private sector. They may be right, but we will have to wait until the smoke of debate clears before we find out. And that might take a long time. So far, at the midpoint of President Reagan's administration, no signals have come from the White House. My own thoughts on this subject are spelled out in Chapter 20.

CHAPTER 13

The GMENAC Report: How Many Specialists Do We Really Need?

ONE FORM of regulation was not tried by the government during the 1970s. No attempt was made to control the delivery system by manipulating the education of doctors. Perhaps this was because medical education was one area where the profession was adamant about its autonomy, where the line had been clearly drawn against government interference. Perhaps it was because the government had already been burned by its programs to increase the number of physicians during the 1960s and now had second thoughts. Or perhaps there were just no guidelines or criteria for the appropriate numbers and types of physicians we should be educating. We have seen that the profession ignored and resisted the government's attempts to increase the number of primary care physicians, especially family practitioners (Chapter 8). Was everyone waiting for the report of the Graduate Medical Education National Advisory Committee (GMENAC) for guidance?

The government established GMENAC in 1976 to advise the Secretary of Health, Education, and Welfare (now Health and Human Services) on the number of physicians required in each specialty, with the idea of bringing the supply of physicians and the demand (requirements was the word the government used) for them into balance. The committee was also supposed to recommend methods to improve the geographic distribution of physicians and mechanisms to finance graduate medical education.

The final report of GMENAC was published on September 30, 1980. It has created considerable controversy but no action to date. How helpful are its answers? Let us look at the concluding statement of the report:

The Graduate Medical Education National Advisory Committee, after three years of intense study, using newly developed mathematical models for estimating the future supply and requirements for physicians, concludes:
  1. There will be 70,000 more physicians than required in 1990.*

---

* The expected entry into practice over the next ten years of 40,000 to 50,000 graduates of foreign medical schools accounts for more than half of the surplus. There will be 145,000 more physicians than required by 2000."

2. Most specialties will have a surplus.*

3. Some specialties will be in balance, including the primary care fields of osteopathic general practice, family practice, general internal medicine, and general pediatrics.

4. Shortages will be experienced in psychiatry, physical medicine and rehabilitation and emergency medicine.

5. Valid criteria for designating geographic areas as adequately served or underserved have not been developed.

Factors contributing to the impending surplus in 1990 are the increase in entering class size of U.S. allopathic and osteopathic medical schools from 8,000 to 19,000 over the past fourteen years, the yearly influx into practice of three thousand to four thousand alien and U.S. citizen graduates of foreign medical schools, and the steadily rising numbers of medical visits cared for by nurse-practitioners, physician assistants, and nurse-midwives.

GMENAC recommends: A 17% decrease in U.S. medical school enrollment compared to current levels; sharp restrictions of the entry into the United States of students from foreign medical schools; no further rise in the number of nonphysician health care providers being trained; and prompt adjustments in the number of residency training positions in individual specialties to bring supply into balance with requirements in the 1990s.

Other recommendations relate to the desirability of increasing the number of minorities in medical school, the urgent need to develop criteria for assessing the adequacy of health services in small geographic areas, initiatives to improve the geographic distribution of physicians, programs to emphasize ambulatory care and training, and new professional service reimbursement plans to help achieve health policy objectives.

The Report will be successful if it generates controversy and improvements. GMENAC is an experiment in policy development through collaboration between the private sector and the government working in open public forum. The collaboration should proceed into its next phase.

On the question of financing, the report replies that hospitalized patients should continue to pay for graduate medical education; that is, teaching hospitals should continue to pay residents' salaries and other costs of their educational programs out of patient revenues. The issue of how to improve the geographic distribution of physicians, however, is left hanging. No recommendations are given because the committee felt there was no way of knowing, "in the absence of valid criteria," whether a specific geographic area was adequately served.

What the report mainly deals with is its primary charge: how to bring supply and requirements into balance for each specialty. The committee developed two new mathematical models, one to estimate supply and the other to estimate the need for physicians in each specialty. As to total number of physicians, the report projects an absolute surplus of 70,000 by

* "Cardiology, endocrinology, neurosurgery, and internists specializing in pulmonary disease will have nearly twice the numbers required."

1990 and a more serious surplus of 145,000 by the year 2000. It seems the American Medical Association was right all along; there is no absolute shortage of physicians, just lopsided distribution into specialties.

The report indicates that if combined private and governmental initiatives are taken immediately, we may be able to balance the system sometime during the 1990s (there is doubt that any change can be accomplished before 1990). If the committee's recommendations are not followed, it may be the twenty-first century before the American people see an end to escalating medical care costs and have easier access to care. But to this reader, *there is no hope in the report that we will ever see an end to the present concentration on treatment, with its ignoring of prevention and health promotion.*

There can be no quarrel with the mathematical model GMENAC used to project the supply of physicians; it was based on sound empirical data. But the method used to determine the *requirements* for physicians is certainly open to criticism by anyone who takes the trouble to read all 800 pages of this seven-volume report.

The requirements model employed a modified Delphi technique, using an expert panel of the specialists and subspecialists in each area. (Delphi panels vote by secret ballot of the individual members on each issue presented to the panel. The outcome of the first ballot is then presented to the panel and the result thoroughly discussed. Individual members give arguments in favor of their viewpoint. Then another secret ballot is conducted. This process is continued until a consensus is obtained. The consensus becomes the panel's judgment.)

The expert panels were asked to estimate, for instance, the number of cases of the most common conditions in their specialty they expect to see, nationwide, in the year 1990. They also gave opinions on such things as the frequency and total number of visits required to give adequate care for each episode of illness for each condition; which tasks and/or visits could be delegated to a nonphysician assistant for each condition treated; and how productive each specialist could be (that is, how many patients a specialist could see in a working day, considering the time that must be spent in teaching, research, and administration).

All these estimates were then put into a computer and out came the requirements for physicians in each specialty for the year 1990. The data put into the computer were, at best, educated guesses by experts. The Delphi technique may be a good way to obtain consensus on a panel, but to know whether the consensus is right or wrong requires faith in an oracle most people don't have.

These doubts about the requirements model are compounded when one discovers that the Delphi panels were often second-guessed by a small number of GMENAC members, not from the specialty in question, called a *modeling panel*. In most instances, the adjusted estimates of the modeling panel rather than the original estimates of the expert Delphi panels were those chosen by GMENAC for its final report. This tactic, of course, destroys whatever validity there is in the Delphi method.

One specific panel, the Adult Medical Care Delphi Panel (made up of members of the various specialties involved in providing primary care), was second-guessed on 50% of its judgments. This panel had been asked to estimate the workload of primary care physicians—including general/family practitioners, osteopaths, and general internal medicine specialists —for the major conditions they would expect to see in patients seventeen years of age and older. When this Delphi panel estimated that primary care physicians would have 199,407,000 visits per year for treatment of obesity, the modeling panel reduced the figure to 36,818,000. Similarly, esimated visits for essential benign hypertension (high blood pressure) were reduced from 117,687,000 to 53,239,000; migraine from 31,114,000 to 4,639,000; and well-care from 99,556,000 to 35,794,000.

The magnitude of these adjustments is so great—in the case of migraine, over 600%—one wonders why GMENAC bothered to use the Delphi panels in the first place. Window dressing? Is the modeling panel omniscient? How could they detect all those "errors" in the judgments of the Delphi panel? Are there reasons for the adjustments other than those given in the text? Does the text lend itself to misreading? After reading it again and again, it is hard to avoid the suspicion that something is wrong. The reasons the modeling panel gives for its changes are quite astounding. Perhaps GMENAC didn't expect anyone to take the time and trouble to read all the volumes of fine print.

Here are some of the reasons for the adjustments given in the text. The report states: "Major changes were made when the reference data and the Adult Medical Care Delphi Panel judgments differed significantly; in such instances, a more intermediate value was chosen." "Reference data" refers to data showing current practice. For instance, the reference data would show how many cases of migraine were currently being seen by primary care physicians and how many by neurologists and other specialists. Since the Adult Medical Care Delphi Panel was estimating the number of migraine patients that would be seen by primary care physicians, not specialists, one wonders if the modeling panel's reduced estimates for migraine encounters shifted treatment to the specialists.

Apparently this was the case, for the report went on to explain: "In other instances, the judgments of more specialized Delphi panels were given preference; *e.g.*, ob/gyn in relation to female genitourinary disorders. In other words, if the Delphi panel of obstetricians and gynecologists said a woman with cystitis (bladder infection) should be seen by an obstetrician or gynecologist, then the modeling panel assigned treatment of cystitis to the specialists rather than to primary care physicians. Does this decision reflect a conspiracy against primary care or a prejudice or just an arbitrary judgment? The next quote rules out an arbitrary judgment: "Reductions in the norms of care for various conditions reflected the modeling panel's judgment that a larger number of visits in 1990 should accrue to specialists or subspecialists rather than to generalists; *i.e.*, more . . . hypertension and ischemic heart disorders to cardiologists, etc."

There it is, out in the open. There can be no question that primary care is getting the shaft; it is being stabbed in the back. Is this a conspiracy against family practice? Were the Delphi panels just an attempt at a cover-up? Why admit to adjustments? (But then, why didn't Nixon destroy his tapes?) Who is behind this report?

Frankly, it sounds like a manifesto for specialists. The report comes right out and says that more people should see specialists than generalists; and more than that, they should see subspecialists if they are available. More people with heart disease, for instance, should see cardiologists, not general internal medicine specialists.

Is this evaluation too harsh? Was GMENAC's motive to give the American people the "best"—always the specialist or subspecialist, with the greatest depth of knowledge in a particular field? But there is an assumption here that is prejudiced and uninformed, and it will lead to an injustice. What is defined as best is not good enough for the American people; we deserve better treatment. It is better treatment to have the most appropriate physician provide care and advice for each encounter that results from each separate and different iatrotrophic stimulus. (Iatrotrophic stimulus is a term coined by Dr. Alvan Feinstein of Yale University to mean any impulse that makes a person seek the services of a physician.)

As I have already pointed out, the most appropriate physician in 80% of these encounters is the primary care physician who has been specifically trained to provide this kind of care and advice—namely, the family practitioner. Dr. Frederick Robbins, dean and professor of pediatrics and community medicine at Case Western Reserve University, goes even further. In his foreword to Jack Medalie's *Family Medicine: Principles and Applications* (1978), he states: "The primary care physician plays a critical role in the health care scene, since he or she can deal with 90% of all patient complaints." In the same textbook, Dr. Lynn Carmichael, chairman of the department of family medicine at the University of Miami, is quoted as saying that in more than 80% of such encounters the condition is self-limited (in other words, no other physician need be consulted).

To have a specialist or a subspecialist provide the care or advice in such encounters is totally inappropriate. Yet this is what the GMENAC report advocates. Most specialists are overqualified and thus not competent to handle these patient complaints. So the quality of care is inferior and the cost excessive, considering the usual fees of specialists compared with family physicians.

This is not to say that we do not need the in-depth knowledge of the various specialists and subspecialists we now have. We do need them, but not in the numbers we now have or in the numbers recommended in the GMENAC report. The committee seems to have been less than candid with the American public. I strongly suspect that the report underestimates the excess of specialists we will have in 1990.

The committee assigned many of these excess specialists to primary care. In determining the mix of primary care physicians, the modeling panel arbitrarily gave everyone under seventeen years of age to the pediatricians, so that pediatricians made up 19% (37,750) of the primary physicians required in 1990. General internal medicine specialists made up the largest number—37% (73,800). Moreover, all osteopaths were assigned to primary care, forming 12% of the total (23,850). The remaining 32% (64,400) consists of family practice physicians and those older general practitioners who will still be active in 1990. These various physicians "assigned" to primary care will make up almost 40% (214,300) of the total (535,750) projected for 1990. Specialists will number 60% (321,450) of all physicians, but the report believes only 70,000 will be in excess of our needs. If we need only 20% of physicians to be specialists (107,150), then the excess of specialists could be in the range of 214,000.

A closer look at the 40% of physicians "assigned" to primary care in 1990 reveals only the osteopaths and the general/family practice physicians as competent and willing to care for the 80% of all encounters that do not need the services of a specialist. Pediatricians won't see adults and many teenagers won't see pediatricians. Internists won't see children, deliver babies, or treat women with "female problems." They will probably refer to other specialists all cuts, scrapes, lacerations, bruises, sprains, strains, fractures, dust in the eye, beans in the ear, runny noses, ingrown toenails, and other conditions of that ilk. Any problem with an emotional aspect is certain to be referred to a psychiatrist.

Yet osteopaths (4%) and family practitioners (12%) together will make up only 16% of the total number of physicians in 1990. Specialists will make up the remaining 84%. Even if we grant that most of the work of pediatricians can be considered true primary care and add the 7% of physicians who are pediatricians to the primary care mix, we still have 77% of all physicians in specialties and only 23% of all physicians capable of providing high-quality primary care. This figure is a much more realistic assessment than the 40% in the GMENAC report.

The modeling panel itself had some difficulty in assigning internal medicine specialists to primary care. In doing so, it loaded the deck, so to speak. Take the matter of productivity. The report admits: "Having established an estimate of total visit requirements for general adult care, it remained to allocate these visits to general/family practitioners vs. physicians in internal medicine. Since the two groups have different productivity, the total head count of required physicians is sensitive to this allocation." Family physicians are nearly twice as productive as internists; they can provide 6,900 visits per year compared with 3,600 for internists in caring for patients needing primary care. We must assume that being sensitive to the differences in productivity meant that the modeling panel had to double the requirement estimates for internists because they were only half as productive. This certainly skewed the requirements.

But it wasn't enough. In dividing the workload between family practice and internal medicine, the report further rationalized the panel's actions: "To make this division, the modeling panel initially assumed that the projected supply of family practitioners will be fully utilized. This assumption resulted in a substantial absolute and relative projected surplus of general internists. The modeling panel, therefore, as part of its continuing function to improve upon its requirements modeling process, apportioned the total number of visits between general/family practice and physicians in general internal medicine, such that the resulting percentage surplus of supply relative to requirements would be equal for the two specialties." If at first you don't like the results, try again.

So, we are faced with a dilemma. Should we throw out the whole report as a conspiracy against family practice, or at least a faulty design of the requirements model, which favors specialists? If nothing is done, we will be left with the present imbalance of specialists, which grows worse each year. If the report is accepted and its recommendations acted upon, it will cast overspecialization in bronze for the rest of this century.

When one realizes that what the report envisions as the time physicians will allocate to "well-care" in 1990 is only time spent doing preemployment and insurance-required physical exams, it is even more discouraging. It forecasts a continuation of the Medical Establishment's nearly exclusive attention to treatment of disease, without concern for prevention and promotion of health.

There must be a better answer. Maybe it is some consolation that in 1990 we will still have the capacity to provide the greatest amount of medical care the world has ever seen—if anyone can afford it.

CHAPTER 14

The Physician of the 1980s: The Fall from the Pedestal

THE REPORT of the Graduate Medical Education National Advisory Committee has given us a reliable mathematical model to estimate the supply of physicians as to the numbers, types, and mix of specialists we will have in 1990 if we continue our present educational policies (see Chapter 13). Even if we were to change that policy today and retrench on the number of specialists we educate and adjust the mix, it would take a minimum of ten years to begin to affect the composition of the profession. And unless we can change the numbers and types of specialists we train, we cannot change the delivery system.

The point is: We are stuck with our present system at least until the mid-1990s. It behooves us then to know how it operates, understand its motivations, and learn how to deal with it. By 1990, there will be at least 70,000 excess specialists out to make a buck (there will probably be a much greater surplus because, as we saw in the last chapter, the GMENAC report undoubtedly underestimated the excess). And, as we learned in Chapter 9, although there will be no need for these 70,000 excess specialists, they will find diseases to treat—at our expense.

How soon we can change the medical care system to the appropriate numbers and mix of specialists and the correct proportion of primary care physicians will depend on how soon the Accreditation Council on Graduate Medical Education acts to adjust the residency programs. And it won't act until the profession agrees that this should be done.

Physicians determine how medical care is provided. They control not only the professional component of the Medical Establishment but all the other components as well. They may not always realize it, but what physicians do or do not do affects the hospitals, the drug companies, and the health insurance industry. Physicians are the core of the Medical Establisment, the center around which the system is built. And, at the moment, the majority appear happy with the status quo.

Some physicians, it is true, are beginning to see the Medical Establishment for what it is—a sickness care machine running out of control.

Not even the profession is controlling it anymore; it seems to have gotten out of hand, everybody's hands. Most physicians, however, seem totally oblivious to the problem. They resent any interference, any attempt to regulate the system, even self-regulation by the profession. They blame any problems—if they find any problems—on the government, the insurance industry, the hospitals, and the "misguided liberals" within the profession, in that order.

It may be easy to understand the attitude of these physicians, but one cannot condone it. It is precisely this aloofness, this inability or unwillingness to see the larger picture, to look beyond their own practice, that has been a major contributor to the problem. Let us take Dr. George Peters, an average American physician.

&ost; In the world of economics and politics, George Peters is a naive and simple man. He does not perceive the consequences of the changes that have been occurring in the system during the last twenty years. There is no deviousness or deceit; he is just a nice guy who would like to be left alone to practice his profession.

"Why should I get involved in the politics of medicine?" he asks. "My expertise is medicine. Let the AMA take care of the politics."

But Dr. Peters is beginning to believe the AMA has let him down. He's known all along that organized medicine, the AMA, is in reality only a small body of politically oriented physicians. It is they who have determined the course of the profession over the last fifty years. Yet, he admits, their stance is conservative; they have tried to preserve the status quo on most issues.

"Everything's all right . . . we have the best medical care in the world, don't we? Why change it? We don't want to throw the baby out with the bathwater."

That's what the AMA says whenever it is threatened with any change, be it Medicare, Medicaid, or a proposal for national health insurance. Dr. Peters is reassured. He'll be able to go on practicing medicine just as he's always done. He even begins to believe that the cry "wolf" is merely a Pavlovian conditioned reflex. He shrugs his shoulders and laughs it off. "It's all politics."

But one morning Dr. Peters wakes up and discovers he is considered the enemy of the poor and elderly. The profession needs a good PR job, a new image, he thinks. He finds out that several of his colleagues have already expressed their displeasure by withdrawing from AMA membership. (At one point in the late 1960s and early 1970s fewer than 50% of individual physicians felt the AMA spoke for them.)

Dr. Peters is almost swayed, but not quite. He hears the AMA's battle cry and falls in line with the rest of the troops. "The politicians are all yelling 'crisis.' Physicians have to unite; they have to stand behind the AMA. If they don't, we may end up with socialized medicine."

Like many physicians, Dr. Peters is haunted by the specter of socialized medicine, a horror story told in chilling detail by the AMA. He himself has had experience with government medicine in the armed services during World War II. He's heard what it was like in Korea and Vietnam. And the stories about medical practice in the Veterans Administration are no better. He wants none of it. Everyone tells him—and he believes it—that national health insurance is the first step toward socialized medicine.

Dr. Peters believes in individual freedom. It is his right to choose his specialty and where to practice, to set his own working hours and his fees for service. And his patients should have the same freedom of choice; they should have the right to choose their own physician.

Dr. Peters also believes he knows what is best for his patients. Whether they realize it or not, he tells himself, we have the best medical care system in the world. Anyone who says we don't must be either a communist or a socialist, or at least a bleeding liberal—a term he had liked ever since he saw a movie in which a Tory made that accusation of a colleague in the British House of Commons.

Dr. Peters is hurt by criticism of himself or the system. It's unfair. Ever since he saved his first life, he has had a sense of superiority, close to omnipotence, which makes him resent fault-finding. He looks at the consumer movement with aloof contempt. Don't they know he is doing his best? Don't they realize that the good he does overrides any temporary inconveniences? What he sees is an attack of his motives and skill; he remains blind to the many inequities developing in the changing system.

The traditional doctor-patient relationship is breaking down, but Dr. Peters doesn't notice this. Like other specialists, he seems unaware that he is becoming more and more distanced from his patients with his insistence on objectivity. He doesn't spend as much time now getting to know a patient; he is less aware of the patient's total personality. And he seems to have forgotten that this can make a difference in treatment.

Often he has an allied health professional handle routine tests and examinations. He doesn't seem to realize that this may create a barrier between the patient and himself. That, whether he intends it or not, the patient may interpret this as a rejection or lack of interest on his, the doctor's, part.

When pressed, Dr. Peters will admit that fewer Americans now have a family doctor who takes an ongoing responsibility for their medical care needs. But, he points out, all his affluent patients have family specialists: They have their internist, gynecologist, allergist, pediatrician, and surgeon. He does, too. Of course he can coordinate the care for his family, choosing the right specialist to match the symptoms of each episode of illness. He forgets that the layperson may not know which doctor is appropriate.

Some of the patients he sees are referred by their internist, who is acting as a family doctor and primary care physician in addition to serving as a specialist. But he's not surprised, or concerned, that 50% of his patients are referred by other patients, not by a physician. Even though he's a specialist, sometimes he hears rumors about other doctors, but he always turns a deaf ear. The stories are just too impossible to believe. Imagine a doctor who is never available after five o'clock and never leaves a substitute on call, so that patients have to use the hospital emergency room at night. What doctor would charge for a telephone referral to a specialist? Or make patients hand over cash for each visit and pay for operations in advance? Someone told him of a doctor who was willing to answer the telephone for only two hours a day, knowing his patients could waste up to two hours of their time trying to get through to him. That's absurd. Nor can Dr. Peters believe that new families moving into town can't find a doctor to take care of them.

Yes, Dr. Peters will admit, many people are forced to use the emergency room as their only source of primary care. And he will acknowledge that usually these people are the less affluent, who can least afford such costly care. But he thinks their insurance will cover the cost. He has no idea what the dollar amount of the charges will be. He hasn't looked at a patient's hospital bill in years. That's the patient's private affair.

Although he is one of those who makes *Medical Economics* the journal most widely read by the profession, he reads only articles pertinent to his personal finances. Tax loopholes and shelters, the advantages of incorporation, sound investments, Keogh plans versus IRAs, how to avoid an IRS audit—that's what interests him. He knows nothing about the economics of medical care.

When he hears about the epidemic of malpractice cases, his pride is hurt. "They're just dumping on doctors." He doesn't see it as a symptom of the profession's alienation from the patient that has accompanied the changes in practice patterns. In his opinion, it's a sign of a growing defect in the character of the American people—at least, some American people. "They want something for nothing; they're after the fast buck, no matter who gets hurt." He also blames the ambulance-chasing lawyers who work on a contingency basis. "Why," he asks, "doesn't someone control the excessive number of lawyers we educate? If there were fewer of them, they would have to stick to honest work. They'd be defending murderers and rapists, instead of picking on hardworking doctors."

If you tell him that America's medical care system is becoming fragmented, inefficient, and impersonal, that it costs too much for most people, you'll be labeled a bleeding liberal. If you recount the problems of access in the inner cities, the storefront clinics, the Medicaid mills, the fraud and abuse in government-financed programs, he may call you un-American. Or he'll say, "That's the government. It fucks up everything it gets into." He can't see his own responsibility in these areas; he is too busy stamping out disease. ੩ॐ

So the average American physician, by not being duly attentive to what has been happening, has inadvertently contributed to the development of what I refer to as the Medical Establishment. A system that no longer relates to the medical care needs of the American people but exists to perpetuate itself. A system that is in love with technology and has lost its human touch. A system that has developed its capabilities far beyond the need for them, that provides unnecessary services just because it is capable of doing so. A system so specialized that it neglects the health of the people, so oriented to the treatment of acute disease that the current epidemiologic revolution, the change to chronic diseases, has passed it by. This system is no longer relevant or even material to the medical needs of the American people.

That is a strong indictment, but it is true. While the system was still germane to our medical care needs, from 1945 to 1975, it produced the golden age of American medicine. Its greatest achievement was to conquer infectious diseases. The system served us well then because it was geared to deal with the acute, short-term nature of infectious diseases. But our needs are no longer the same. Today, the American people require a system that can deal with chronic, long-term illnesses—heart disease, cancer, stroke, and so on. Yet the system has not changed; it approaches these chronic diseases as if they were acute illnesses. Most of the research funds from the National Cancer Institute are spent searching for an "antibiotic" to cure cancer; little is being done to eliminate cigarette smoking, the cause of 90% of lung cancer. The Medical Establishment's approach to coronary heart disease is bypass surgery; it doesn't try to prevent it in the first place. These are just a few examples. We now know how to prevent 50% of our current diseases; yet the Medical Establishment spends 96% of our health care dollars on treatment and 4% on prevention and the promotion of health.

Organized medicine, the most important component of the Medical Establishment, has lost control. It has been more concerned with preserving its eminent position, its economic and political independence, than with leading the profession in a world of rapid social, technological, and epidemiological change. The AMA has not realized that change *is* the status quo, that whatever stands still is already obsolete and will be left behind.

Most physicians still do not see the danger ahead. They don't realize that as they become increasingly alienated from those they are dedicated to serve, they may no longer be attending to patients' real needs. More and more, they may find it will become easier to slip over that fine line where they have stopped serving people altogether and have begun using them to serve their own ends. This would be the ultimate immoral act. It is what happened to Adam Americus.

Perhaps a fall from the pedestal we have been placed on for three-quarters of a century will shock us into a soul-searching reevaluation of our value system as a profession. We must begin by changing the way we choose candidates for admission to medical school. We must put a premium on people-oriented individuals and encourage young physicians to enter the field of primary care as family practitioners. We must, as a profession, begin to appreciate and respect the family doctor as the ultimate example of the ideal physician. Finally, we must design our delivery system to meet the medical and health care needs of the American people.

CHAPTER 15

Warning: Medicine Is a Two-Edged Sword

THE MEDICAL ESTABLISHMENT has the ability to provide us with the best in medical care. But, as we have seen, for 80% of our medical needs, it is overequipped and the physician is overqualified. Consequently, we are often overtreated.

This overtreatment is particularly dangerous because medicine is a two-edged sword. Every drug, by its nature has a toxic effect (although sometimes this may not appear until the next generation). Every procedure carries the potential of death; every operation risks complications. And hospitals can be very dangerous places; unless it is essential to be there, stay out.

The Medical Establishment knows these dangers, but it pays them little heed. It continues to define "best" as "most." The result is that, in general, the less contact you have with today's Medical Establishment, the less will be the risk to your health.

Take X rays but don't take them lightly. It is not like having a photograph taken. The effect of X-radiation is cumulative over one's lifetime. Although it will never add up to the amount of irradiation that the people of Hiroshima and Nagasaki received, a small dose can have grave consequences. Only now are we beginning to see thyroid cancers that are the result of treating acne and enlarged thymus glands by X ray over thirty years ago. And recently, we have begun to realize that mammography, another X-ray technique, may cause more breast cancer than it ever detects.

X-ray and especially the new computerized tomography (CT) techniques are important and necessary diagnostic tools. They can save lives. But we should reserve X-ray exposure for these livesaving needs. Unfortunately, one-third of all X rays today are taken defensively, out of a fear of malpractice suits on the part of physicians. This expensive and dangerous practice is a sad commentary on our contemporary system.

Another realm of abuse is medication. Many of the drugs prescribed today were unknown ten or even five years ago. Each year a physician receives a new copy of the *PDR* (*Physicians' Desk Reference*), which lists all the prescription drugs currently available. Scores of new drugs are added each year. (Ask your doctor if you can look through his copy the next time you are waiting in his office. Chances are that he will be using it himself; he can't keep all this information in his head. You may have better luck in your local library.)

Many of the drugs being prescribed have not been used long enough to know what the toxic effects may be. Take diethylstilbesterol (DES), which was prescribed for pregnant women to prevent miscarriage during the postwar baby boom of the 1950s. Many of these women's female offspring are now developing cancer of the genitalia. (The congenital defects in their sons' genitalia showed up much earlier.)

Little did we know that the wonder drug tetracycline would permanently discolor the teeth of children who received it. The drug has also been deposited in their bones; what long-term effects this will have, we still don't know. We didn't know that another antibiotic, streptomycin, would cause deafness or that chloromycetin would depress the blood-forming tissue of the bone marrow. We didn't know that butazolidin, a drug used in treating arthritis, could cause leukemia or that the contraceptive pill might lead to hypertension, heart disease, liver tumors, or cancer of the uterus. And we didn't know that aspirin, which so many people take without thinking, could interfere with the blood's clotting mechanism, leading to hemorrhage. We didn't know. We didn't know. We didn't know!

Every procedure of an invasive nature, whether it involves puncturing the skin with a needle or entering an orifice with an instrument, carries the danger of infection. And infection is the least dangerous complication; an acute allergic reaction called anaphylactic shock, cardiac arrest from a nerve reflex, even death, can result.

Every operation has a mortality rate. In many cases, the greatest risk comes from the use of a general anesthetic. This risk is about 0.1%—but for that one person in a thousand the mortality is 100%. If one in every thousand airplanes that took off were destined to crash, most of us would travel by train.

My point is that nothing in medicine should be taken lightly. There is always a risk. And the risks must always be weighed against benefits. Fortunately, with much medical care today the benefit outweighs the risk. Take appendicitis, for example. The risk of the operation, 0.1%, is negligible compared with the risk of not removing an acutely infected appendix and letting it rupture, which is 5% to 10%, depending on the age of the patient. Even removing a few normal appendixes—up to 20% is considered good practice—to avoid letting one rupture and cause peritonitis is less risky. But in many areas of contemporary medical practice this is not the case; the risk is too great for the benefit. Our armamentarium—the contents of our little black bag today—is truly wondrous, and in some cases these weapons against disease can be lifesaving. We should be thankful we have them when we need them. But to use them just because they are there, or to use a complex procedure on an elementary problem (an elephant gun to kill a mouse), is irresponsible and dangerous.

Swept away by its love affair with technology and all it can now do, the Medical Establishment no longer always serves the best interests of the American people. In the next three chapters we will look at three classic examples of how the Medical Establishment's dedication to "progress" has led it astray. For instance, treatment may be provided for the benefit of science or knowledge, not for the patient. In some cases, people have become the latest breed of laboratory animal, however unwittingly. Cancer chemotherapy (discussed in Chapter 16) is one illustration of this kind of abuse. A different, but equally questionable practice of our contemporary Medical Establishment is its overreliance on surgical procedures that may not be necessary. In the Prologue, I described the rush to aorto-coronary bypass grafting. Another telling example is the rapid rise in Caesarean sections, which has resulted in a higher maternal mortality rate, with no significant improvement in mortality rates of the newborn (see Chapter 17). A final example of how current practice has gotten out of hand is the way end-stage renal disease is treated (see Chapter 18). The Medical Establishment's "kidney heroics" provide a clear instance of how the system may do something just because it is technically capable of doing it. It doesn't seem to matter that neither society nor the individual benefits from the expenditure of health care dollars or the robbing of the medical commons.

CHAPTER 16

Human Guinea Pigs and the Poison Doctors: The Dangers of Research

IN 1971, Congress declared war on cancer. If our Research Establishment was given enough money, it was felt, the cause and cure of cancer could be discovered in our lifetime.

It is now ten years later, and the war is being lost. More of us are contracting the diseases—cancer is not one disease but several—and more are dying from them than ever before. Cancer of the lung has taken the lead, causing 117,000 deaths last year. Although the incidence of others, like cancer of the stomach, is declining, it is not because of a victory on the research front. More than likely, the decline, in stomach cancer at least, is caused by a change in diet.

The war is directed from Washington, D.C., by the National Cancer Institute (NCI), while the battles are fought in twenty comprehensive cancer centers throughout the country. The battlefields include such renowned institutions as M.D. Anderson in Houston and Memorial-Sloan Kettering in New York. But NCI is calling the shots. So far, the leaders have advanced only one strategy—the search for a magic drug, the "antibiotic" for cancer.

NCI's minions hope to discover drugs that will selectively kill tumor cells but have little or no effect on normal cells. So far, they haven't found any. Yes, they have found some that affect tumor cells more than normal cells. But the risk of damage to normal tissues far outweighs any benefit from these drugs. Yet NCI persists in its testing. There seems to be no end to the number of chemicals that can be tested. And there seems to be no end to the number of human guinea pigs who can be used.

The research gods, however, seem to be growing angry; they seem to be turning their backs on NCI. The research gods are very touchy beings who guard their mysteries well. Rarely do they reveal their secrets to mere mortals, and then only in small bits and pieces, never in one big revelation. Revelations come by serendipity to conscientious researchers as rewards for their diligence; it may be that the gods have become frustrated watching someone go down a blind path for too long, and so they send a beam of

light. Honest researchers realize that their insights are not always the result of logical deductions or inductions on their part. Discoveries seem to
occur when least expected. And although the researchers are usually unaware that the gods have befriended them, they do call it luck.

NCI is undoubtedly out of favor with the research gods. No serendipitous revelations have occurred, and none is likely as long as NCI continues its *directed* research. Directed research rules out serendipity. In
directed research, only experiments that follow one predetermined line of
reasoning are funded. No one can go off on a tangent to explore a lead,
hither and yon, wherever it goes. Researchers must stick with the one
designated approach if they want to be funded. NCI has kept its troops in
line, even though its soldiers realize the war on cancer is being lost.

There is hope, however, in the provinces, where guerrilla forces have
been waging more successful battles. Denied funds by NCI, they have had
to live from hand to mouth. But they have been diligent and steadfast,
and the research gods have smiled on them. There have been several
serendipitous breakthroughs. New weapons, especially immunotherapy in
combination with surgery and chemotherapy using the older and safer
drugs, seem to be extraordinarily successful. The guerrillas have begun to
glimpse victory in sight.

Still, on the larger, official front, the fighting continues without question. Nor does NCI appear to be alone in its blind faith in chemotherapy.
There is a whole new breed of specialists in medical oncology (the non-
surgical treatment of cancer), who look for the day when they can wrest
the treatment of cancer from the hands of the surgeons who have controlled the field so far. Surgeons now refer to this group as the *poison
doctors.* Yet the use of chemotherapy—the systemic administration (usually
intravenously) of chemicals in the treatment of cancer—is still in the experimental stage. In all honesty, it should not be looked upon as treatment
but as a type of continuing research, a clinical trial.

The specific chemicals chosen for this clinical testing come from many
sources, from natural substances like weeds that poison cattle to synthetic
chemicals like ballpoint pen ink. Most are extremely toxic; they have to be,
since they are expected to kill living cells. These chemicals are first tested
on laboratory animals, usually mice with leukemia, to see if they kill tumor
cells without killing the mice. Next they must be tested on humans because
a drug may behave differently in man than in a laboratory animal.

The first tests on humans are called Phase I studies. The purpose of
these tests is to determine the toxicity of the drug in humans. What are
the side effects? What is an appropriate dosage? These studies are *not*
done to see if there is a therapeutic effect on the tumor. The dosage first

tried on humans is only one-tenth the amount that killed 10% of the mice. But this amount is rapidly increased in an attempt to determine the maximum sublethal dose in humans.

It is in the Phase II studies (usually limited to one research institution) and Phase III studies (usually cooperative studies involving several centers) that the effect of the drug on human cancer is evaluated. The results are measured in partial remissions (in which 50% of the tumor cells are destroyed) or complete remissions (all tumor cells) of temporary or lasting duration. Clinical judgment enters into these evaluations. Much is subjective, leaving room for variations depending on the investigator's enthusiasm or prejudices.

But where do they find the human volunteers to test these various chemicals? It's obvious; they choose patients with cancer, especially those who have not responded to conventional cancer treatment methods: surgery, radiation, and commercially available chemotherapeutic agents of relatively low toxicity (Methotrexate, Cytoxin, Vincristine, Adriamycin, Bleomycin, and Cisplatin). The low-toxicity anticancer drugs are credited with "curing" (that is, arresting the disease, with no recurrence for five years) somewhere between 11,000 and 46,000 cancers a year, according to estimates by Dr. Vincent DeVita, the director of NCI. Although these statistics include the combination of chemotherapy with surgery and irradiation, chemotherapy can be said to contribute to the cure of between 1.5% and 6% of the over 800,000 cases of cancer seen in the United States each year. Surgery cures about one-third of all cancers and radiation another 5% to 10%.

It is the six out of ten cancer victims who are not cured by these current methods of treatment who become the eager guinea pigs for clinical trials. When you have been told you have a deadly disease and there is no assurance that you have been cured by the proven methods, you are willing to try anything that offers hope of cure or postponement of death, even for a short time. I know. I've been there. I had my left lung removed for cancer four years ago. As a physician, I knew that only 10% of lung cancer is cured by conventional measures.

How exactly do these clinical trials work? Most clinical trials use a different protocol for the various stages of cancer. All malignant tumors are staged by the profession in making a final diagnosis. Staging is an attempt to indicate how advanced the disease is in a specific individual. The size and microscopic appearance of the tumor itself is referred to as T; whether or not it has spread to local or regional nodes is noted under N; and spreading (metastasis) to other parts of the body is graded under M. Staging permits more accurate evaluation of the various types of treatment, determination of the most appropriate treatment, and more accurate prognosis. It prevents comparing apples with oranges. Stage I (written T_1, N_0, M_0) carries the best prognosis because it means that the tumor is small, localized, and has not spread beyond the organ of origin. (My cancer was Stage II: T_2, N_1, M_0.)

In all this, we must not forget the primary purpose is testing. The guideline is research, not treatment of the patient per se. Clinical trials are the only means of evaluating the efficacy of various methods of treatment, for comparing the results of surgery versus irradiation versus chemotherapy, or a combination of one or more modalities. Each treatment variation may be tried as a separate "arm" of the protocol. For the patient willing to participate in the clinical trial, the arm of the protocol he or she receives is chosen by random selection. The idea is to prevent adverse selection by the patient or the investigator and thus make the experiment more objective.

Such clinical trials are considered an ethical form of human experimentation because the patient gives informed consent and the efficacy of any one of the protocol arms is unknown at the time. No one is simply being used as a control in the experiment—the control "treatment" may prove to be the most efficacious. And the potential benefit of any new treatment method or drug usually outweighs any disadvantage in the participant's mind since nothing else has worked. It is like playing Russian roulette, but you are willing to grasp at any straws.

Still, there are questions we need to ask. In October 1981, the *Washington Post* published a four-part exposé on chemotherapy clinical trials. Entitled "The War on Cancer: First Do No Harm," the articles were written by two staff reporters, Ted Gup and Jonathan Neumann. As a result of their investigations, Gup and Neumann challenged not only the medical ethics of this kind of research but also the humaneness of the methods used. They ask if the physician's oath to "first do no harm" has been upheld in the use of these experimental drugs. Specifically, the *Post* investigators found:

While all anticancer drugs can cause side effects among some of those who take them, the experimental drugs—in addition to leading to hundreds of deaths—have elicited a nightmarish list of serious adverse reactions, including kidney failure, liver failure, heart failure, respiratory distress, destruction of bone marrow so the body can no longer make blood, brain damage, paralysis, seizure, coma, and visual hallucinations.

So little is known about many of these chemicals that doctors have found these ironic results: In some cases the experimental drug actually stimulated tumor growth rather than stopped the cancer; and in other tests, doctors and researchers found that the experimental drugs themselves caused cancer.

In many cases, the experimental drugs have been given to patients even years after studies failed to show that they were of use in the fight against cancer. The first phase of the experimental drug program, in fact, is primarily designed not to combat cancer, but to find out how toxic the drugs are.

Physicians at some of the nation's leading hospitals and cancer centers have inadvertently administered high or miscalculated doses of these potent toxins with fatal results.

Records of some drug experiments have been so poorly kept that dates of patients' deaths are off by months, lab reports are lost or never done, and responses to drugs are misrepresented. In addition, some hospitals and the NCI have in written reports exaggerated the therapeutic performance of the drugs.

Drugs and treatments not approved by the FDA for human use—and not authorized by the NCI—have been administered to dozens of patients.

The litany of death and suffering from experimental drugs has become an accepted part of life at some hospitals around the nation. These human experiments have gone largely unchallenged and unquestioned by Congress, the medical profession, and the scientific community at large. How and why did it reach this point?*

I was lucky; I refused to participate in the first clinical trial I was offered. Intellectually I didn't like the choices and emotionally I wasn't ready to leave my future to chance. Generally, as a gambler I had always been a loser; it seemed that this was the prudent time to walk. My surgeon agreed that he would have done the same thing.

But I owe my life to another clinical trial, which I was lucky enough to be able to participate in. I had served on the Commission on Cancer of the American College of Surgeons for nine years; I was an insider. Through friends, I made contact with Ariel Hollinshead, head of the Virus and Cancer Research Laboratory at George Washington University. She has developed a vaccine against certain forms of cancer, using tumor-associated antigens that she isolated from the cell membranes of cancer cells. She directed me to Dr. Tom Stewart at the University of Ottawa and his associate Dr. Jules Harris at the Rush Medical School in Chicago, who were doing a clinical trial with her lung cancer vaccine. I was subsequently admitted to their Canadian protocol and received the chemo-immunotherapy arm of that study.

It has been over four years now, and I am alive and well and free of cancer. I am in the process of reclaiming my own life.

The story of Ariel Hollinshead, a woman scientist in our Research Establishment, and her struggle to obtain funds for her research while the NCI continues its myopic search for an anticancer drug—well, that is the subject of another book.

How would I advise a friend or loved one faced with the dilemma of

* Ted Gup and Jonathan Neumann, "The War on Cancer: First Do No Harm."

whether or not to participate in a clinical trial? I would say to first ask a lot of questions or have a physician you trust ask them for you. If they can offer hope of a cure, if others have had a complete remission, then I would say yes. If the best they can offer is palliation, if no one has had a complete remission, then I would say no. Your chance of living longer under these conditions is negligible, and chances are the quality of your remaining time will be much better without chemotherapy. If they are only offering a Phase I study, run for your life.

Clinical trials, however, may be the only way we will discover new ways to combat cancer. Properly used, they are an ethical form of human experimentation and should continue. But the individual who participates must be honestly and completely informed as to what is in store for him or her in consenting to the experiment.

Any gain for society that results from the uninformed submission to such experiments is immoral. On the other hand, there is no greater love than participating in such clinical trials if one is aware of the risks. But this means that the medical profession must cull from the many only those experiments which can truly benefit society, knowing they may be balancing this gain against the cost of a human life.

Even more devastating, however, is the current practice of giving incurable cancer patients chemotherapy just because there is nothing else to do. No clinical research is involved but the doctor feels helpless and therefore suggests chemotherapy knowing that no one has ever been cured by this particular "treatment." My advice here is the same: If they can offer hope of a cure, if others have had a *complete* remission, then I would say yes. Otherwise, say no.

CHAPTER 17

Caesarean Section:
For Love of Technology and Fear of
Malpractice Suits

A CAESAREAN SECTION is a surgical incision through the abdominal wall and uterus, performed to extract a fetus at, or just before, full term. The name comes from the Latin word *caedere*, "to cut." It is said that the ancient Roman name Caesar derives from one born by this procedure— *a caeso matris utere*, "from the incised womb of his mother." Legend tells of Julius Caesar himself being born in this manner.

Esther, the elderly midwife, is beginning to sweat. Her wrinkled skin is moist, but her mouth has grown dry. She turns her head to wet her parched lips on a damp upper arm; her eyes, however, remain fixed on the moribund young woman who lies on the straw pallet, unconscious now, her skin blue-white, covered with moisture, scarcely breathing.

A moment before, her face was red, purple-red. Her scream of pain still rings in Esther's ear.

A recurring wave of nausea breaks over the old woman; the stench has grown worse. Urine, feces, the bag of waters that broke the day before, all have soaked the straw—waftage now in the heat, suspended, except for a momentary breath of air from the one small window near the ceiling.

Esther looks up. The sky is becoming light again—the second dawn since labor began. A cock crows and the dogs raise their impatient whines to howls, waiting for the afterbirth.

They know, she thinks. 'Twill be the funeral pyre that gets the afterbirth this day.

She hears the men pacing in the next room. The unsteady clop of their boots on the marble floor had echoed throughout the night. For a time, though, the sound had stopped, and she had smelled the musky incense from the shrine of the household god. Then later, much later, came the bleat of a sacrificial lamb and the stench of burning flesh. They, too, know, she thinks.

The two young female slaves cower together in a corner; they are of no help. Throughout the night she had prayed to her god, Jehovah, for the life of this young mother and her firstborn child. Why hadn't He heard?

Esther is a free woman now, a citizen of Rome. The best midwife in the city, they say. She is always in demand for the noble ladies. This one's father is a senator, from the ancient Roman family of the Julii, and her husband is a centurion, from another branch of the same family. But citizen or not, she knows if there is no child to expiate for this mother's death, her own life will be in jeopardy. And if the child is female, her fate may be the same.

She puts her hand on the belly; how cold it is. The womb hasn't contracted now for several minutes. She slips her other hand between the lips and feels the cervix, still hard and thick over the baby's head. She puts her index finger in the anus and feels for the head. It is still high, tight against the bone; it hasn't moved in hours.

She bends her ear to the woman's belly. Is there any sound? Is the baby alive? She isn't sure. Ah, there is movement. A kick. Life!

She picks up the knife and wipes it clean on her skirt as she always does just before she cuts the cord. "Oh, that you should only have to cut a cord," she whispers to the blade.

The cock crows again. The dogs are yelping now, and the boots beat an impatient cadence.

"Deliver me, Lord," she prays. And, with a swift stroke, she slits the belly up the middle from pubes to breastbone.

She cuts through the gut. Its green liquid mixes with the dark-red blood—an evil omen. No matter. She sweeps it aside and lifts the womb.

The knife cuts into its dome. Scarlet blood—a better sign. Then, a gush of water that has been trapped by the baby's head.

She pushes two fingers into the hole and cuts between them, down as far as she can. A spurt of blood hits her face; she can't see.

But she feels one foot, then the other. She drops the knife and wipes her face on her upper arm. She pulls both legs, and the small body unfolds. But the head doesn't budge. She twists the torso like a corkscrew. Finally, the head is free.

Now she slaps the baby's bottom. There is no cry. Again she slaps. And again.

She forces her little finger into the baby's mouth and removes the white amniotic curd she finds.

Again she slaps.

Now she places her lips over the tiny face and softly blows life into the child.

It shudders. A gasp. Then, a cry. What a glorious sound.

It is a boy. Only now has she dared to look.

She weeps. And then she laughs as her own urine runs down her legs into the straw. ❧

In those days the procedure was used only *in extremis*—to save the life of an unborn child of a dying mother, usually one unable to complete delivery because the infant was too large for the birth canal. Roman law permitted the practice.

The first known instance of a Caesarean being performed to save a woman's life occurred around 1500. A Swiss gelder of pigs is said to have used his knife on his wife when delivery was blocked. She lived, but the procedure remained dead for several hundred more years.

The first successful Caesarean section in the United States was also performed by a man on his wife. Dr. Jesse Bennett operated on his wife, Elizabeth, near Edom, Virginia, long before the operation was accepted as an obstetrical procedure. Dr. George M. Nipe, writing recently in *Virginia Medical*, tells of the physician's heroic effort to save his wife and child.

On January 14, 1794, Elizabeth began labor with her first pregnancy. Labor was obstructed, probably because of a contracted pelvis. The widely known veteran obstetrician, Dr. Alexander Humphreys, was summoned from Staunton to consult. Forceps delivery was attempted without success. Craniotomy was then advised, but Mrs. Bennett refused to accept the death of her child to save her own life. Caesarean section was then proposed by Bennett, but Dr. Humphreys refused to perform an unknown, potentially dangerous procedure. He returned to Staunton when it was obvious that this was the only solution acceptable to the young mother.

Many hours of labor had passed by this time and it was no doubt abundantly evident that immediate action was necessary. Jesse Bennett decided to operate on his wife at once.

The patient was given a large dose of opium and laid on a table of planks supported by two barrels. Two Negro women aided the doctor. The initial incision opened the abdomen and uterus. The child, a living female, and the placenta were delivered . . . the uterus and abdomen were closed with linen sutures. To everyone's amazement, Mrs. Bennett recovered, apparently without serious complications. The child lived to be 77 years of age.*

* G.M. Nipe, "Jessie Bennett Decided to Operate on His Wife at Once."

Dr. Bennett is thus credited with the first successful Caesarean section performed in America. Mrs. Bennett was lucky, for during most of the following century the recorded mortality was about 75%. Few physicians had the courage to attempt Caesareans. Instead, craniotomy, the crushing of the fetus' head to permit passage through the birth canal, was usually done in an attempt to save the mother's life.

Only at the end of the nineteenth century—after the introduction of antisepsis, improved surgical techniques, and better anesthesia—did Caesarean section become an acceptable alternative to the sacrifice of the infant by craniotomy in cases of arrested labor or other complications of normal vaginal delivery.

Today, Caesarean section (usually referred to as C-section by the profession) is a relatively safe procedure. For the last two decades, maternal mortality has averaged about one in 1,000 C-sections. Still, until 1960, only 4% to 5% of deliveries were accomplished by this means. It was not considered an elective alternative to vaginal delivery. It was used only when there were complications of labor, and only with specific indications —when experience had shown that a C-section would be less dangerous than permitting the mother in labor to continue to try to deliver vaginally.

Beginning in 1960, however, the frequency of Caesarean births began slowly to increase. By 1970, the rate had doubled. In the last ten years, the incidence has tripled in the United States (an increase not seen in other countries).

Hospital Utilization Project (HUP) data from 240 U.S. hospitals, for the period from July to December 1980, place the incidence at 19% of all births. In some institutions, a rate of 25% to 50% is not uncommon. And in some quarters of the Medical Establishment, C-section is being touted as the new wave, the "normal" birthing method of the future.

Other physicians disagree. They state that the increase does not represent more accurate diagnosis or better management of problems leading to healthier mothers and babies. Women's organizations are especially upset. They claim that the sudden increase is based on nonmedical factors that are not in the best interests of the mother and her child. They cite such factors as convenience for the physician, increased revenues for the physician and the hospital, and sexist attitudes in a male-dominated profession. A real controversy has developed.

I believe the increased use of the C-section is a striking example of what is happening to contemporary health care under a Medical Establishment caught up in its love affair with technology. The same trend is occurring in many other areas of medical care. Increased technology is increasing costs, increasing risks, and alienating the patient, without any real improvement in outcome and frequently with a deterioration in the patient's health.

Even conscientious physicians appear to be trapped in a system that seems more concerned with its own well-being than with that of the patient. It is essential for our future health that we look at all the facts in this development and that we question the Medical Establishment.

Why the sudden increase in C-sections, for instance? Are more American women requesting Caesarean birth?

No! Most women today seem to prefer natural childbirth. Birthing units in hospitals are being furnished with only an old-fashioned bed, home deliveries are becoming more popular, husbands insist on being with their wives during labor, and nurse-midwives are becoming a new type of health practitioner.

Has there been an increase in the classical indications for Caesarean section that would justify an increased use of the procedure?

No! The classical indications for C-section have been generally accepted, without debate, for the past fifty years. They consist of mechanical problems caused by a disproportion between the size of the baby and the size of the birth canal in the mother (*cephalopelvic disproportion*) or by the position of the baby in the uterus (*malpresentation*); problems involving the placenta, which attaches the umbilical cord to the wall of the uterus, like the roots of a tree to the earth, and through which the fetus is nourished from the blood supply of the mother; and medical problems of the mother that make labor and/or vaginal delivery dangerous to her or her child.

Cephalopelvic disproportion is the primary mechanical problem. It can be caused by a small, contracted pelvis in the mother or a large head on the baby, or both. The baby simply cannot pass through the birth canal, it becomes stuck, and labor cannot progress normally.

Malpresentation is another indication of a mechanical nature. Normally, the baby's head enters the birth canal first (*presents*) and, during labor, the head's round shape molds and stretches the birth canal as the baby descends, dilating the cervix (the open end of the uterus that protrudes into the vagina). If any part of the baby except the head presents, this shape may be inadequate for dilating the birth canal and labor does not progress. The most common malpresentation is when the buttocks presents; this is called a *breech*. The shape of the buttocks, basically similar to the head but smaller, usually will allow the birth process to proceed normally. But if a foot, arm, or shoulder presents, the umbilical cord may well get caught between the baby and the wall of the uterus, and this would cut off the blood supply to the baby.

There are two abnormalities of the placenta that may require a C-section. The placenta can be attached to the uterine wall at the cervical end, where it blocks the opening of the uterus (*Placenta previa*). Or there can be a premature separation of the placenta from the wall of the uterus during labor (*Abruptio placentae*). Both of these conditions can result in fetal death owing to lack of blood supply before the baby has a chance to breathe on its own and thus to oxygenate its own blood.

A C-section is also indicated when certain medical conditions in the mother make labor dangerous. Diabetes and hypertensive states associated with toxemia of pregnancy usually call for early abdominal delivery. Certain infections in the mother, especially those of the cervix or vagina (e.g., herpes), may contraindicate a vaginal delivery.

However, none of these classical indications has increased in incidence in the past fifteen years. What, then, are the indications being used by the profession to justify the more frequent use of this procedure?

Actually, there is one other classical indication—a previous Caesarean. This indication has been the leading cause of the increase in C-sections since 1916, when the doctrine of "once a Caesarean, always a Caesarean" was first promulgated. By 1960, it had become the indication for 30% of all Caesareans.

In 1916, there was good reason for this rule. The procedure then in vogue, called the classical section, cut into the top of the uterus, lengthwise, in its midline (the most thinned-out portion of the wall at term). In subsequent labors, this scarred area was prone to rupture with the uterine contractions, with catastrophic consequences. Elective C-section was therefore indicated before labor began. (This practice, incidentally, led to more premature infants, who have a higher threat of complications and require more specialized care—frequently by a neontologist, a pediatric specialist in the care of the newborn.)

In the early 1960s, however, this method of performing a Caesarean was replaced by a crosswise incision made low on the thicker part of the uterine wall. With a scar in this area, there is only a remote possibility of rupture with subsequent labors (about 1 per 1,000). Consequently, the old doctrine is no longer applicable, *yet it is still being used as an indication.* According to Dr. S. Bottoms and his colleagues, writing in the *New England Journal of Medicine* in 1980, this indication has been responsible for 23% of the increase in C-sections since 1960. It is now the indication for 40% of all C-sections.

The indication that is causing the largest increase in the C-section rate, however, is *dystocia* (33.4%, according to Bottoms et al.). This new, catchall indication includes not only classical cephalopelvic disproportion but also functional difficulties that produce a slowing or arrest of labor. "Failure to progress in labor" or "uterine inertia" are the new buzz-terms that reflect this shift in thinking from a purely mechanical to a functional approach. These functional causes for arrest in labor are frequently iatrogenic—physician-induced. The use of fetal monitors, pitocin drips to induce labor (IV drip of drug causes contraction of the uterus), and premature rupture of the membranes (bag of waters) can all lead to uterine inertia.

Labor graphs, a new technique for monitoring fetal heart rate and uterine contractions, are used to confirm the diagnosis of dystocia. Less reliance is placed on pelvimetry (ultrasound visualization of the size of the baby's head relative to the pelvis). But is it appropriate to make this decision to do a Caesarean on the basis of labor graphs alone?

Obstetricians openly state that their goal is no longer to achieve a vaginal delivery. It is more important to have undamaged infants, and thus they should allow only a reasonable duration of labor, not prolong it. The words sound noble and compassionate. But the devil's advocate could ask: Can't this also be interpreted to mean that if you haven't bothered to do pelvimetry, don't fret? With your new monitors you can get tracings that will justify a C-section after a "reasonable" period of time. No need to stay up all night or try too hard for a vaginal delivery; get on with the C-section.

Breech presentation is causing 18.8% of the increase in the rate of C-sections, according to Bottoms et al. It's not that there has been an actual increase in breech presentations, however; what has changed is physicians' attitude toward delivery of a breech. (Remember the difficulties Charlie faced in Chapter 8.)

C-section is the ultimate remedy for any complication that might occur from a breech or other malpresentation. But what is happening is that obstetricians are not waiting for the complication to occur. They are moving the patient into the operating room as soon as the diagnosis of a breech is made. They feel that the risk of doing a C-section is less than the risk of a malpractice suit for not using the ultimate remedy. (Those who thought they might make a buck by having their lawyer sue the physician for minor and unintentional mistakes of omission or commission have to share in the blame for this one.)

Furthermore, this indication is self-perpetuating. As fewer vaginal deliveries are done with breech presentations, the resident in training has less experience with this alternative to the C-section. Together, this gap in physicians' education and the current malpractice climate are leading the new generation of obstetricians to abandon the vaginal breech delivery.

The situation has developed without any clear proof that C-section improves the outcome for all breech-born infants. In fact, there has been no significant decrease in perinatal mortality (death of an infant within the first twenty-eight days of life, excluding those that weigh less than 1,000 grams) among breech-presenting infants delivered by C-section compared with those delivered vaginally.

The fourth major indication, accounting for 13.2% of the increase, according to Bottoms et al., is *fetal distress*. The marked increase in this indication has paralleled the increased use of fetal heart rate monitors. It might even be concluded that fetal monitoring is the cause of this indication. Does this mean that before fetal monitors were introduced we didn't know when the fetus was in distress? It might seem so, but it is not the case. If it were, there should be an improvement in perinatal outcome in this group of infants. But no improvement has occurred, despite the high rate of C-sections. In addition, there has been no reliable correlation between abnormal monitor tracings and other measures of fetal distress, such as the pH of fetal scalp blood. In fact, in one center, when they would not accept the monitor's diagnosis of "fetal distress" without first checking fetal scalp blood pH, they reduced the rate of C-section from 24.4% to 11.7%.

So what is the value of a monitor that appears to be so inaccurate? At best, it is probably reliable only as a warning signal for possible fetal distress. At worst, it is an iatrogenic cause of more Caesareans. The monitor generates stress in the mother, leading to the release of catecholamines (adrenal hormones) into her blood, causing constriction of the blood vessels and thus reducing the blood flow through the placenta from mother to child. All this affects the baby's heart rate and indicates distress on the monitor.

Fetal monitoring can also increase the incidence of functional arrest of labor (dystocia) by interfering with uterine contractions. When hooked up to the monitor, the expectant mother is forced to be inactive and to stay in a horizontal position. The chance of dystocia increases because she cannot walk about during labor. The situation is further complicated when a pitocin drip is running. Too large a dose of pitocin may lead not only to uterine inertia but also to fetal distress.

Then why do obstetricians continue to rely on monitors? The only rational explanation seems to be the blindness that frequently accompanies a love affair with technology. It would, of course, be blasphemous to the god Technos not to show respect for a scientific instrument, not to rely on what it tells you but instead use your own good judgment.

The threefold increase in the rate of C-sections has brought concomitant benefits to the Medical Establishment. Revenue has increased, tertiary care institutions are put to greater use (C-sections help to pay for the high overhead), and staffing is more efficient (less personnel is needed around the clock). For the physician, there is also greater convenience, less threat of malpractice, and a higher income. One assumes these benefits are the result, not the cause, of this trend.

Consumers, however, may take a different view. They pay higher fees and higher insurance premiums. Often they are handled in an assembly-line manner, and are alienated from their physicians. Moreover, they are deprived of the unique experience of normal childbirth.

What about the socioeconomics of the matter? C-section nearly doubles the length of stay (LOS) in the hospital. The average LOS for 20 hospitals, according to HUP data for July to December 1980, was 3.7 days for vaginal delivery and 6.7 days for C-section—3 extra days. Total hospital charges also increase. In one Chicago hospital, thirty of the hospital's own employees (or dependents) were delivered during the six months ending in March 1981, and 33% were Caesarean births. For the twenty vaginal deliveries, the average LOS was 3.2 days and the total charges were $2,313; for the ten Caesareans, the average LOS was 5.4 days and the total charges $4,626 (exactly double the cost). And this figure does not include the fees of the obstetrician, the anesthesiologist, or the neonatologist in this tertiary care institution.*

Even if we assume that all the socioeconomic benefits to the Medical Establishment are only byproducts of this practice, there are other questions that must be asked. Is this trend to more and more Caesareans safe for the mother and her baby? Is a Caesarean just as safe as vaginal birth? Are obstetricians justified in making the act of childbirth more scientific? Are there any benefits?

Obstetricians point out that the perinatal mortality rate has shown a marked decrease over the past fifteen years, paralleling the increase in C-section. Cause and effect? Probably not.

H. Minkoff and R. Schwartz found a positive cause and effect relationship only when mechanical obstruction (cephalopelvic disproportion) was the indication for the C-section. Moreover, they point out, other improvements in obstetrical and pediatric practice can also be credited

---

* Many insurance programs will pay for a C-section even when their usual coverage excludes normal childbirth. There is no evidence, however, to show that this situation has caused an increased use of C-section.

with a lower perinatal mortality. They conclude that "it is difficult to justify the precipitous rise in operations on the basis of better outcome." L. Mann and J. Gallant, of the University of Vermont, agree. "We cannot conclude that these improvements in perinatal outcome are a direct result of a more liberal use of Caesarean section."*

What about maternal mortality? Is the risk to the mother increased over vaginal delivery? A recent task force report issued by the National Institute of Child Health and Human Development, National Institutes of Health, claims that the mortality for Caesarean delivery is four times as great. Other studies claim that in some geographic areas it is almost thirty times as great. For instance, J. Evrard and E. Gold, in their 1977 study of 160,000 births throughout Rhode Island, found a maternal mortality rate of 2.7 per 100,000 vaginal deliveries and 69.5 per 100,000 C-sections (twenty-six times higher). In 1980, however, F. Frigoletto et al. reported that 10,231 C-sections were performed at Boston Hospital for Women (a tertiary facility associated with Harvard Medical School) without a single death, although the maternal mortality rate for vaginal deliveries was 10.27 per 100,000.

So much for statistics! Where lies the truth?

Peter J. Huntingford of the London Hospital Medical College asked the same question in the *Journal of Biosocial Sciences* in 1980. Noting that the increase was largely an American phenomenon, he wondered if he and his British colleagues had missed the Mayflower. He writes:

If the increase in Caesarean sections in the U.S. is due to better medical practice, or the result of more accurate diagnosis and better management of problems leading to healthier mothers and babies, then there would be a case for a comparable rise in Caesareans in Britain. However, if the U.S. rise is due to other, nonmedical causes, a corresponding rise here would not necessarily be justified. It would not be the first time that operations have been carried out unnecessarily on a large scale and the error discovered only years later. One recalls the large increase in tonsillectomies which began in the late 1920s and persisted at a high rate for thirty years until an outbreak of poliomyelitis in the 1950s led to the postponement of many operations and finally to the realization that, for the majority of children, the operation was not needed.

After studying Caesarean births at twenty hospitals on Long Island, Huntingford concluded that the British should not follow the American trend. He stated quite candidly that it would not be in the best interests of women or their babies. Referring to the monitors and other new techniques used in these hospitals, he remarked: "Innovations in medical

* H. Minkoff and R. Schwartz, "The Rising Caesarean Section Rate"; and L. Mann and J. Gallant, "Modern Indications for Caesarean Section."

technology are used indiscriminately without proper evaluation so that instead of increasing diagnostic accuracy they lead to more surgical intervention."

Huntington also addressed the problem of the individual confronting the Medical Establishment: "It is an unusual woman who in the middle of labor can challenge medical advice, especially when it is apparently based on objective evidence and accurate electronic observations." He also raised the question of sexism, asking: "How much of the increase is due to the need for male obstetricians to retain control of a process in which they cannot otherwise participate so that they remain dominant?" He concluded: "We believe that the increase . . . can be accounted for by nonmedical factors that protect the interests and authority of the medical profession over women."*

Most American physicians would take umbrage at such statements. But my own observations as medical director of a large teaching hospital and my extensive research on the subject lead me to conclude that the alarming increase in Caesarean births is caused by physician-generated, technological, and medical-legal factors—not medical indications.

My advice to a woman who would like to avoid an unnecessary Caesarean section is relatively simple. First, take responsibility for your own body and your baby's. Read and become well informed about the whole process of pregnancy as well as delivery alternatives. Attend prenatal classes with your husband and ask questions about anything you don't understand. Choose your obstetrician from those whose C-section rate is 6% or less. Choose your hospital from those whose rate is less than 10%. (There is a higher correlation between choice of obstetrician and the likelihood that you will have a C-section than between the choice of hospital and that likelihood.) Ask about hospital policies. What percentage of deliveries are monitored? What are their policies on rupture of the membranes to initiate labor and use of pitocin drip to augment labor? How many hours can you be in labor after your membranes rupture before they demand a C-section? Ask your obstetrician these same questions. Also ask about breech presentations. Does your obstetrician believe all breech presentations should have a C-section? What is his or her position on "once a Caesarean, always a Caesarean"?

Remember that we have the best medical care system in the world—if it is used intelligently, in partnership with an understanding and compassionate physician. Under these circumstances, hospital delivery is

---

* C. Francome and P. Huntingford, "Births by Caesarean Section in the United States of America and in Britain."

much safer than home birth. If you prefer a nurse-midwife, be sure she is supervised by a reliable obstetrician. If you prefer natural birth, choose an institution with a birthing unit, so that immediate backup facilities and services are available in case of complications.

Involve your family physician. If he or she has obstetrical privileges in a good hospital, you are probably in the best of hands. If not, have your family physician advise you in choosing an obstetrician and hospital—but still ask your own questions. Use your family physician as your advocate in confronting the Medical Establishment. Never forget that it is your right to ask for a consultation or second opinion if you have any doubts.

But also remember: There are definite indications for a Caesarean section that can save your life and that of your baby. Develop a trusting relationship with your physician—or choose a different one.

CHAPTER 18

Kidney Heroics: Who Benefits?

IN 1972 Congress enacted a piece of legislation that has since come home to haunt it. It was during the expansionist era of our health care delivery system, and the legislators wanted to assure that more and more Americans would have access to needed medical services. It was Congress' first —and probably last—attempt to cover a categorical disease, that is, to provide care for individuals with a specific health problem (in this case, kidney failure). What resulted was an inadvertent experiment that has almost guaranteed that we will never see comprehensive national health insurance legislation passed.

Specific diseases have from time to time caught the interest of segments of the public, and people have formed voluntary private organizations to concentrate the fight against the particular illness. Funds have been raised to promote research into the cause and cure of the disease or to pay for the treatment of victims. Many groups were started because a loved one of the founder or a prominent individual contracted the disease. The March of Dimes, for instance, was a tribute to Franklin Delano Roosevelt's fight with poliomyelitis. Lou Gehrig's illness spawned the group fighting the neurological disorder amyotrophic lateral sclerosis. The American Heart Association, the American Cancer Society, and many other well-known organizations speak to the concern of individuals in the private sector.

But never before had Congress attempted to sponsor one specific disease. It had covered segments of our population, broad categories of our people, with programs such as Medicare for the elderly and Medicaid for the poor, but never this.

Perhaps this legislation passed because Congress was tired. It was attached to Social Security amendments that had been in the legislative hopper for four years. When Senator Vance Hartke (D.–Ind.) put forward his proposal, there were already numerous other amendments designed to improve Medicare and Medicaid. It was September 30, 1972, at the end of the 92nd Congress, and there was little time for debate. Perhaps Hartke was eloquent in his support, or maybe he hit an emotional note, sounding a responsive chord in his peers. "How do we explain that the difference between life and death in this country is a matter of dollars?" he asked. Whatever the reasons, the end stage of a primary disease of the kidney—end-stage renal disease (ESRD)—became a covered service under Medicare with the passage of P.L. 92-603.

The intentions of the sponsors of this legislation appeared to be honest and good. They wanted the technique of hemodialysis for kidney failure to be made available to young individuals who were otherwise healthy, allowing them, because of this treatment, to return to active, productive lives.

Hemodialysis was developed in 1960. When an individual's kidneys fail to function, an artificial kidney machine is used to cleanse the blood of the toxic products of metabolism, the impurities that form as the result of muscles contracting, the heart pumping, and other organs carrying out their normal functions.

In the early days of dialysis, the patients were young, mostly in their late thirties. Kidney transplantation, using close relatives as donors, was known to be successful, and techniques for using other donors, including kidneys from recently deceased people, were being perfected. It was reasonable that these young people, who sometimes had to wait for over a year for a suitable donor, should not be allowed to die for lack of funds before a transplant could be performed.

At the time, the annual cost of dialysis was $40,000. Few young people or their families could afford this expense. Hartke was sincere. "How do we explain that the difference between life and death in this country is a matter of dollars?"—especially when we were already nearly a trillion dollars in debt. What were a few more bucks when lives were at stake?

By 1980, however, the few more bucks was adding $1.2 billion a year to the cost of Medicare. Five percent of Medicare's budget was being spent on 0.2% of the eligible beneficiaries (about 57,000 individuals). And only a few of these 57,000 resembled the young person Hartke had envisioned—someone waiting for a transplant so he or she could be rehabilitated and return to work. Today, the average age of a dialysis patient is well over fifty. Only about 3,500 will ever receive a transplant, and most have no prospect of returning to work. In fact, most are permanently disabled and are receiving disability payments from Social Security that amount to an additional $300 million. This expense raises the total cost of the ESRD program to $1.5 billion per year.

But the cost is only one problem with the program. Moral and ethical problems have developed that cause greater concern. The end-stage renal disease program has become just that, an end-stage program.

Before dialysis, when an individual's kidneys failed, when they stopped putting out urine, death was inevitable. In a few cases, however, the kidney failure was only temporary, for instance, in acute poisonings or shock following injury or surgery. In these cases, dialysis by peritoneal lavage could occasionally keep the patient alive until the kidneys recovered and began working again. Peritoneal lavage consists of placing large quantities of water into the abdominal cavity and allowing the lining membrane, the peritoneum, to act as a filter so that the impurities pass from the blood into the lavage water; in essence, acting as a substitute kidney.

Peritoneal lavage, however, provides a very inefficient kidney. Even the original synthetic kidney was much more efficient. The artificial kidney circulates the patient's blood outside the body, through plastic tubes, like cellophane, that act as semipermeable membrane filters. These tubes are immersed in a water bath. The ions of highly concentrated impurities, dissolved in the blood plasma, pass through the semipermeable membrane into the water, where the concentration of ions is lower (solutions on either side of such a semipermeable membrane, which allows ions to pass through it, tend to reach an equilibrium in their concentration of ions). The blood, freed of its impurities by this means, is then returned to the patient in a continuous cycle. Hence the name hemodialysis for this process.

A single hemodialysis treatment usually takes three to four hours. If repeated three times a week, it reaches the efficiency of an individual's normal kidneys. Barring complications, this procedure can keep a patient alive indefinitely.

Consequently, artificial kidneys quickly replaced peritoneal dialysis. Until the development of kidney transplantation, hemodialysis was used only in the treatment of temporary kidney failure. The possibility of transplantation, however, made hemodialysis essential. It was necessary until a donor could be found, and, should a transplant fail, the patient had to be returned to dialysis until another transplant could be arranged. If this was not possible, then the patient had to be maintained on dialysis for the rest of his or her life. Today, this result is less frequent with young people because of the increasing success of transplants using cadaver kidneys.

According to S. D. Roberts et al., writing in the *Annals of Internal Medicine* in February 1980, individuals with end-stage renal disease, that is, in the end stage of a primary disease of the kidney, assuming their other organs are healthy, can expect nine additional years of life because of the ESRD program. If they had to pay for these nine years out of their own pockets, it would cost them $168,000 apiece in medical bills over their remaining lifetime. (And no one I know would deny them the ESRD funds to pay for this.)

ESRD patients have four options for treatment. If they can find a close relative to donate a live kidney for transplant, their life expectancy will increase to 14 years. With a cadaver transplant, life expectancy is 8.2 years. They may also choose to forgo a transplant and continue with hemodialysis. If they do this at home, they can anticipate 9.5 years of dialysis; if they choose a center for dialysis, their life expectancy will be 8.4 years.

The quality of the ESRD patient's life will be much better with transplant, especially from a living related donor because he or she will need less immunosuppressive therapy to prevent rejection of the transplanted kidney. Dialysis patients, on the other hand, have many psychological problems; divorce rates are about 50% and there is a sevenfold increase in the rate of suicide.

The government would prefer that ESRD patients choose a live, related-donor transplant because the cost to the ESRD program is lowest: $7,709 per life year. Home dialysis next, at a cost of $13,274; then cadaver transplant, at $14,918. Center dialysis, either in a hospital or freestanding, is the most costly, at $24,800 per life year. The government estimates that the program would save $284 million per year if there were a shift from center dialysis to either home dialysis or cadaver transplant.

Kidney failure, however, is also an end stage of many chronic diseases: cancer, heart disease, stroke, hypertension, and just plain old age. In many cases of chronic illness, the kidney happens to be the vital organ that fails first, instead of the liver, heart, or brain. These terminally ill individuals are also entitled to dialysis under the ESRD benefits of Medicare. And instead of being the exception, this type of patient is rapidly becoming the norm.

It has reached the ludicrous stage where senile patients are being transported across town three times a week from their nursing home beds to a dialysis center for treatment. There are documented cases in the states of Washington and Massachusetts where the families and physicians of these incompetent individuals have asked to have the dialysis stopped but have been forbidden to do so by the courts.

Fortunately, most of these legal standoffs have been solved by the patient's death, but the dilemma remains. Dialysis has become the latest life-support system, and until the patient's heart stops or the brain dies— a new and additional legal definition of death in most states—no one has the guts to pull the plug!

Perhaps we are fortunate that kidney transplants were developed before heart transplants. Can you hear someone in Congress now asking colleagues, "How do we explain that the difference between life and death in this country is a matter of dollars?" Had we all been entitled to heart transplants, including the right to be kept alive until we could have one, in some end-stage cardiac disease program, then we would already have seen the day when we were spending all of our gross national product on health care. All of us would have to live on life-support systems because all of our money would be allocated to keeping us "alive"; there wouldn't even be money left to bury us.

Ridiculous? Certainly. But how far are we from ridiculous in the end-stage renal disease program?

Soon after the ESRD program was enacted, I was asked by the California Regional Medical Program to serve on a task force to develop a quality assurance program for end-stage renal disease. I was elected chairman of the group, perhaps because I had written two books on quality assurance—one for hospital care and another for long-term nursing home care. We all assumed that the criteria for quality of care that the task force developed would be used by the Department of Health, Education, and Welfare in writing regulations for the ESRD program. But it wasn't. Had HEW used just our first criterion—"It should be assumed that everyone admitted to the program is a candidate for kidney transplant"— it would have prevented the problem the program faces today.

Those working in dialysis programs have severely criticized the government for not writing sufficient regulations for implementing the legislation in the first place. There are also complaints of inadequate leadership, a management information system that has yet to provide useful feedback, and the habit of passing the buck when problems arise. No one seems to be in charge. "If this is what we can expect under national health insurance," they say, "we want none of it."

Very few in the program today are candidates for transplant. Hemodialysis has become an end in itself. It has become a big business; indeed, those in the for-profit, proprietary business of dialysis appear to be functioning very well in the absence of government regulation of the program.

There are approximately 1,000 dialysis units in the United States. One-third are located outside hospitals, and most of these (75%) are run for profit. About 50% of all dialysis patients, however, are treated in these freestanding units. About 10% of patients are on home dialysis and the remaining 40% are dialyzed in hospitals.

In the early years of hemodialysis, 40% of patients were on home dialysis, the least expensive alternative for the patient. But in the ESRD program there is a financial drawback for patients on home dialysis. They have to pay for supplies out of their pockets—supplies that would be paid for by the program if they were dialyzed in a unit. It's not surprising, then, that many have given up home dialysis.

The largest proprietary dialysis company is National Medical Care, Inc. It has cornered 17% of the dialysis market and appears to be the most powerful force in the field today. NMC is listed as the largest operator of dialysis centers and, as of December 31, 1980, had 137 outpatient centers in twenty-one states and Puerto Rico. In many cities it is the only option available. Its stock is traded on the New York Stock Exchange. NMC also owns a subsidiary, Erika, that makes all its dialysis equipment and supplies. Moreover, it has its own laboratory to do the lab work for all NMC patients.

The ESRD program accounts for 77% of NMC's revenues. The NMC second-quarter report for June 30, 1981 showed revenue for the first half of 1981 of $139,461,000 (up 21% from 1980) and a net income of $11,736,000 (up 4%). NMC's assets are listed at $229 million and its stockholders' equity is $104.9 million. And NMC expects a 60% increase in the number of its patients by mid-decade. (It is not known whether this increase will be caused by a higher incidence of renal disease or NMC's having a larger share of the market. My broker couldn't tell me.)

Like the ESRD program itself, NMC had innocent beginnings. In the early 1960s, Dr. Constantine Hampers, now chairman of the board, and Dr. Edward Hager, now chairman of the executive committee of NMC, were nephrologists in Boston. They were in charge of the dialysis unit at the Peter Bent Brigham Hospital, one of Harvard Medical School's most prestigious teaching hospitals. According to Gina Bari Kolata, writing in *Science* in April 1980, these physicians were concerned because, with the scarcity of equipment and the high cost, they frequently had to decide which patients to put on dialysis and which to leave to die. It was natural that when they were asked to become the medical directors of a proprietary extended care facility (nursing home) in 1966, they incorporated dialysis in the plans for the facility. Two years later, NMC was incorporated. By 1970, they had two dialysis centers in addition to the nursing home. In 1972, then, when Congress enacted the ESRD program and thereby guaranteed payment for dialysis treatment, NMC was in a good position to take advantage of the rapidly expanding market.

HEW set a fixed rate of $138 per dialysis treatment in 1973. A hospital-based dialysis unit could ask for a higher reimbursement if it could show higher costs (under the cost reimbursement mechanism for hospitals in the Medicare program). Since most hospitals could show higher overhead, reimbursed costs in hospital units averaged $159. For freestanding dialysis units, however, the $138 rate did not change until the end of 1981.

This payment scheme, incidentally, served as an unintentional experiment in case rate reimbursement. It showed that when physicians know they will only be reimbursed a set amount for a specific treatment, they can be motivated to be more productive, more efficient, and still make a profit, especially if they can share in any savings. NMC's profits from the ESRD program are a good example.

Dr. Hampers is quite proud of his company's performance in this experiment. In a recent article in the *New England Journal of Medicine*, he states: "The success of the ESRD program in expanding service to meet demand while controlling costs and maintaining quality has been due primarily to the combined effect of setting a price and creating a system of incentives that involve physicians in the medical marketplace."*

Perhaps the government read his article and his last-quarter report. In December 1981, the Department of Health and Human Services announced that it was establishing new and lower rates for dialysis under the ESRD program: $133 per dialysis in hospital-based facilities and $128 per dialysis in freestanding units. There will also now be more incentive for home dialysis, because the payment will be the same whether the dialysis is performed in the home or in the unit.

NMC will have to tighten its belt. The physicians who are medical directors of NMC units may not be able to make the $400,000 a year they are reported to earn—at least not for the next year or two. But after that, they should soon be back on target. It is anticipated that the lower rate of reimbursement in the ESRD program may force some marginal units to fold. These units might even consider selling out to NMC. Also, many hospitals may decide to close their units if they are no longer cost-reimbursed. NMC might win the game of monopoly by default.

Will someone in HHS finally write the necessary regulations for the ESRD program? Will Congress finally make it known how it intended

* E. Lowrie and C. Hampers, "The Success of Medicare's End-stage Renal Disease Program."

this Medicare benefit to be used? I wouldn't count on it. NMC has John Sears, Ronald Reagan's former campaign manager, as its lobbyist in Washington.

If I were you, I would buy NMC stock. It was running around $13 a share the last time I looked. That's a price/earning's ratio of 9.3, and Wall Street is projecting a price of $75 somewhere between 1984 and 1986—a 475% gain.

You'll probably need all that money to buy medical care by then.

CHAPTER 19

Maneuvering the Medical Maze: The Need for a Patient Advocate

So FAR, I have suggested that you stay as far away as possible from the Medical Establishment when you are not sick. In the next part you will find out how to avoid being sick—that is, how to stay healthy. But how do you deal with the Medical Establishment when you *are* sick?

All of us get sick from time to time in our lives. It may sound contradictory, but it is a good idea to establish contact with the medical care system before you get sick, even though you are not planning to use it immediately. It is like looking for the nearest fire escape when you check into a hotel, or taking part in the lifeboat drill on board ship. As I was taught as a boy scout, be prepared.

One of the first things you should do when you move to a new town is to find a family doctor. Preferably, you should have your previous doctor call another physician he knows and respects in your new location or recommend someone from the *Directory of Medical Specialists*. This guide lists all physicians who are board certified by their specialty and the community in which they practice. It details each physician's training, experience, and hospital appointments. Yet how a physician performs is another matter. Ask your new neighbors about your choice's reputation around town, this is usually a reliable indicator. While you are about it, check out the reputation of the hospital with which your prospective physician is affiliated.

Try to find one of the new specialists in family practice. Since there are not enough of them to go around, however, you may have to select a general internal medicine specialist. If so, try to choose one who limits his or her practice to primary care.

The next step is to see if this physician is taking new patients. The good ones are usually in demand, but they are also conscientious and will try to accommodate you. A referral from your previous physician will carry weight under these circumstances. When you phone, insist on talking to the doctor in person; don't let an office assistant or secretary take a message. Have the new doctor call you back if necessary, but be sure to mention your previous doctor's name. Just say, "Dr. Smith asked me to call Dr. Perry." Don't say what it is about until you are talking to the doctor directly.

If you can't find anyone to take you, you might try the local county medical society. Since most of these societies are on public record as denying a shortage exists, they will guarantee to find you someone. Another method is to find a good subspecialist if anyone in the family has any special problem. You might, for instance, call a gynecologist and say you need a pap smear—this is usually inexpensive and you probably need one anyway. Once you are in this subspecialist's hands, let him or her find you a family doctor.

After you choose someone, make an appointment for an initial, get-acquainted visit. Most physicians who take on primary care responsibilities like to do a baseline evaluation of your health status at the start. Be sure to take your old medical records with you.

What should you expect? A new doctor will take a complete medical history, perform a physical examination, and do some basic laboratory studies.* Make sure you have your height, weight, and blood pressure checked and that you are tested for glaucoma (tension of the eyeball that can lead to blindness). Men over fifty should have a rectal examination to rule out abnormalities or to detect early cancer of the prostate gland. Men and women over fifty should have a sigmoidoscopy (visual exam of the rectum and lower colon) and a stool examination for blood to rule out cancer of the gastrointestinal tract. Women should have a breast examination and a pap smear to identify early breast or cervical cancer. A skin test (PPD) for tuberculosis should be done and, if positive, a chest X ray. Laboratory tests should include: a hemoglobin (especially in women) to rule out anemia; a urinalysis as a screen for kidney disease; and a cholesterol, high- and low-density lipoproteins and triglycerides analysis for atherosclerosis, and a VDRL for syphilis.

The reason these tests are important is that they rule out the very few diseases for which early detection can make a difference in outcome, both medically and economically. Glaucoma, diabetes, high blood pressure, syphilis, tuberculosis, and some cancers (especially breast, cervix, colon, and prostate) can all exist for some time without causing symptoms. Most other serious diseases are symptomatic early in the course of the illness.

This brings us to the subject of the annual physical, a medical ritual

---

* It's also wise to review your immunization history with your new family doctor. Adults rarely need booster shots except for tetanus, which should be repeated about every ten years.

that is nothing but that—a ritual. It is certainly not cost effective, nor is it medically useful. An annual physical exam is simply a search for signs of asymptomatic disease. To a physician signs are the objective findings from a physical exam or lab test that indicate the probable presence of disease. An elevated blood sugar level, for example, may be a sign of diabetes before the symptoms of the disease become evident.

All the important asymptomatic serious illnesses can be detected by the tests listed above. In addition, these tests measure certain risk factors that are determinants of health (see Chapter 23). It is unnecessary, and may even be dangerous, to submit to a whole battery of tests unless you have specific symptoms. And keeping the tests to a minimum will save you about $300.

You've gone for your initial visit to your new doctor. Now, let's consider subsequent office visits. The average American sees a physician five times a year for routine (nonemergency) conditions. A single visit can cost $50, especially if pharmacy bills are included—and most office visits wind up with a prescription being written. (Unfortunately, many patients feel slighted if they don't have this little piece of white paper in their hands when they leave.) We would all be better off spending the $50 on some healthful form of recreation, since 70% of these visits are probably unnecessary.

But how can one tell which visits are unnecessary? "If I knew it wasn't serious, I wouldn't go," you say. "And sometimes just being reassured is worth $50. I'd rather not take a chance." True, but there is another way.

During our "crisis" in primary care, when physician assistants and nurse-practitioners were being trained to be thrown into the breach as extensions of the physician, a technique was developed to teach them how a physician approaches the diagnosis and treatment of disease. This technique employs an algorithmic approach to decision-making. A series of alternative actions is taken, with each successive choice being determined by the preceding step. This "decision tree" approach has been simplified so that the average consumer can determine in which illness, or when in the course of an illness, a physician should be consulted.

The best guide, especially if you have no training in health care, is *Take Care of Yourself: A Consumer's Guide to Medical Care* by Drs. Donald M. Vickery and James F. Fries. This book contains about sixty-eight decision tree flow charts for common conditions that usually take patients to doctors' offices. It describes appropriate home treatments and when they are safe to use. It also includes a home pharmacopia of drugs that can be purchased without a prescription.

Emergencies, of course, are another matter. Time is of the essence in any life-threatening condition. You should immediately contact the emergency services set up in your community. In most areas of the country, a telephone call to the Operator or dialing 911 will bring an ambulance and trained paramedics to the scene right away. Don't waste valuable time trying to reach your family doctor, although make sure he or she is informed as soon as possible.

(Ironically, Mayor Daly of Chicago, who was responsible for setting up one of the nation's best emergency networks, tried to climb the stairs to his family doctor's office while he was experiencing his fatal heart attack. He became a statistic, one of the 60% of coronary victims who never make it to the hospital.)

In some emergency situations, you cannot even wait until the ambulance and paramedics arrive. The brain cannot live if it is deprived of oxygen for more than a few minutes. Do you know what to do if someone you love is choking on a piece of meat at dinner? Can you simultaneously apply mouth-to-mouth resuscitation and external cardiac massage until the ambulance arrives if your spouse's heart stops from a coronary occlusion or an electric shock? Anyone can learn cardiopulmonary resuscitation (CPR) and other lifesaving first aid techniques at courses given by your local Red Cross or community college. Sign up!

For other, less life-threatening emergencies, such as severe lacerations, hemorrhaging, or fractures, you might simply take the patient directly to the emergency room of your local hospital, rather than call an ambulance. Hospital emergency rooms are designed to handle these crises. More and more hospitals now have physician specialists in emergency medicine staffing the facility twenty-four hours a day.

But emergency rooms should be reserved for true emergencies; they should not be used as the family doctor. It is extremely wasteful and expensive to use emergency facilities for primary care. Moreover, the emergency room physician usually has very little interest in nonemergency conditions. The facility is not equipped to provide follow-up care, so there is no continuity of care. A patient who misuses the service will probably have a long wait and receive short shrift—and pay a lot for it.

Familiarizing yourself with both the emergency and the routine sources of medical care is well worth the effort. It will pay dividends when you do need help. You will have established an ongoing relationship with a family doctor. Although your family doctor may not be able personally to provide all of your future care, he or she is the best guide to other specialists and subspecialists when they are needed. But, most important, you will have a patient advocate in your dealings with the Medical Establishment.

A patient advocate is becoming essential in our fragmented, over-specialized, and highly technical system. You need someone with your interests at heart to guide you through the maze of services and personnel—sometimes just to interpret the language.

Many patients, trying to find their own way, have innocently picked the wrong kind of specialist. Remember what happened to Joe with his ingrown toenail. A woman I knew thought she should see a urologist for her backache. After multiple tests, including an IV urogram, a retrograde pyelogram, and a cystoscopy for which she was hospitalized, the urologist told her he was happy to report that she did not have any urological problems. "It must be your back," he said. "You better see an orthopedic surgeon." She was incensed and $1,000 poorer—but much wiser.

You should use your family doctor as your adviser whenever you are confronted with medical decisions you do not fully comprehend. Suppose a surgeon suggests an operation. Should you follow this advice? If you aren't sure, ask your family doctor to talk directly with the surgeon. Your doctor may agree with the surgeon's advice and then explain why he or she believes you should have the surgery. But if there is any question in your doctor's mind *or in yours*, arrange to get a second opinion from another surgeon.

Never hesitate to ask for a second opinion or a consultation. If the first physician objects, you are better off in the hands of another doctor.

❧ About two years ago, I became hoarse. I went to see a local ear, nose, and throat (ENT) specialist. He found a polyp on one of my vocal cords and recommended surgery. The advice seemed reasonable, but I also understood that, especially in dealing with another physician, the ENT specialist might not want to take any chances and, therefore, was giving me the most conservative advice. I wanted a second opinion.

I went to see Dr. Bill Fee, the ENT chief at Stanford Medical School. He confirmed the presence of a polyp, but he thought it was probably benign since it was located in an area on the vocal cord where malignancy is very rare. In his opinion, the polyp might have developed from violent closing of the cords in response to gastric acid regurgitated, as I slept, into my throat from a hiatal hernia of my stomach.

What he did was to offer me a choice. I could have the polyp removed. Or, if I agreed, I could try taking an antacid at bedtime and sleeping on two pillows to prevent the regurgitation. He would be willing to watch the polyp and see if the prescribed treatment allowed it to regress. I chose to avoid the surgery. In four weeks the polyp was gone, and it has not recurred. ð➤

On the other hand, don't go overboard. Don't force your doctor into arranging for unnecessary second opinions or consultations. You shouldn't blindly follow the advice you get on this or that test from friends over the bridge table. Step over that sleeping dog.

➤§ Ted is an internist in Pennsylvania. He is one of the good doctors I told you about—a people-oriented internist who practices like a family physician. (Whenever I criticize internists in general, I feel badly because of Ted. But then, if all internists were like him, I wouldn't be criticizing them.)

Ted has a patient whom I will call Mabel Smith. Mabel has had a small fibrous tumor (fibroadenoma) in her left breast for about ten years. It is one of those that is near the surface, easily palpated, and characteristically benign. It hasn't changed in size or appearance in ten years.

But one day, while Mabel is playing bridge, she discovers that she is the only one at the table that hasn't had a mammogram. North, South, and East—they've all had one.

On her next visit to Ted she asks, "What's a mammogram?" Ted explains that it is an X ray of the breast used to screen for malignancy in women with large breasts who have had a family history of breast cancer.

"Shouldn't I have one?" she asks.

"No," replies Ted. "Studies have shown that in women with average-sized breasts, physical examination by palpation is more accurate than mammography in diagnosing breast tumors. Your breasts are easy to examine and there is no family history of cancer. Your fibroadenoma hasn't changed in ten years. Besides, I don't want you to have any more X-ray exposure than you absolutely need."

She persists. "I had a great aunt who died of breast cancer. I think I'd feel better if I had one."

"Okay," Ted finally says. "I'll arrange it."

Mabel has her mammogram, and the report comes back: "suspicious of malignancy." Ted is surprised and examines the mammogram results himself. The radiologist indicates that although the tumor is probably benign there is some calcium in the adenoma, and under these conditions he has to label it "suspicious."

Ted calls Mabel in and tells her about the report. He gives her the name of a surgeon.

"But what do *you* think, Ted?" asks Mabel.

"I think it's what I have always said it is—a benign fibroadenoma."

"Well then, we'll watch it." She rises to leave.

"No, we won't." Ted stops her. "Now we have a piece of paper that says 'suspicion of malignancy.' We have to have it removed. I could be wrong. We can't take the chance."

She is operated on. It turns out to be a benign fibroadenoma after all. But she develops a wound abscess, which leaves her with a deformed breast and a large scar (making subsequent examination of her breast difficult). Now, when Mabel plays bridge, she doesn't talk across the table. ?❧

The helpfulness of having a patient advocate can't be stressed enough. And the best patient advocate is your family physician, who has come to feel about you as family because of a long and close relationship. Physicians' families and their close friends are lucky—they have a built-in patient advocate—and most of them seem to need one when you realize that the medical experiences of these families seem to be governed by Murphy's Law (if anything can go wrong, it will). Still, I'd like to cite another example from my experience to underline just how important it can be to have someone to call on for advice when you're faced with a medical crisis. Some years ago I was able to help my daughter through the medical maze. It may have saved her life.

❧ We are at home in California, playing bridge with another couple on a Sunday night. The telephone rings; it's Dick, our son-in-law, calling from Chicago. He and our daughter Ann—who is three months pregnant with her first child—have just been in an automobile accident.

They were on their way to O'Hare Airport to catch their return flight to San Francisco. Dick was driving his mother's two-door coupe, with his father in the other front seat, and his mother and Ann in back. He slowed to turn off the Kennedy Expressway at the O'Hare exit. The ramp traffic was stalled, bumper to bumper. Dick glanced in the rearview mirror and saw a pickup truck bearing down on them. There was no place to turn. He blew his horn and pumped the foot brake. But the truck driver didn't see the flashing lights; he rear-ended them at fifty-five miles per hour.

In forty-five seconds their car was in flames. Burning gasoline spread in all directions on the roadway. How they all got out of the car they don't quite remember. Ann recalls crawling on all fours to escape the flaming gasoline, squeezing under the guard rail, and rolling down the embankment of the ramp. She couldn't walk. She had to drag her right leg—her hip had been dislocated during the impact.

They were taken by ambulance to Resurrection Hospital, a 440-bed, JCAH-accredited teaching hospital, affiliated with a medical school. It is listed in the *American Hospital Association Guide to the Health Care Field* 1980 as having an organized emergency department. The central dispatcher of Chicago's emergency medical services network decided that this was the hospital best able to receive accident victims that night, even though they passed two other excellent hospitals on the way.

As Dick describes it, Ann is the only seriously injured person there. Yet other people in the emergency room, with relatively minor injuries, are being treated and discharged. Ann is still lying on a table; nothing has been done for her hip. There is only one physician on duty, and he doesn't seem to know what to do for her. It is almost midnight, three hours since the accident, and Dick decides he can't wait any longer. That's when he telephones me, his father-in-law, his patient advocate.

I tell Dick to put the emergency room physician on the phone. I explain that I am a physician, a surgeon, and ask what is wrong with my daughter.

"We don't know yet," he replies, describing the situation in broken English that I have difficulty in understanding. He is a foreign medical graduate, a resident in training at another Chicago hospital, who has been hired by Resurrection to cover their emergency room that night. (Although such moonlighting is frowned upon in most residency programs, the practice is still frequently used to cover the night shifts in hospitals that do not have their own house staff. In this way, a resident can earn extra money, over and above a resident's stipend.)

"Haven't you X-rayed her?" I inquire.

"No, she is pregnant and we didn't want to take any chances with the fetus."

"Good God, man, don't you have any lead shields you can put over the abdomen? All you need is a single view to make the diagnosis. Have you called an orthopedic surgeon to see her?"

"Yes. He said to wait until morning—to put her in traction and he'd see her then."

"Look," I said, "if she has only broken her hip, that's okay. But if it's dislocated, it has to be reduced as soon as possible. The longer it is out of the socket, the greater the chance of losing the blood supply to the head of the femur. I want you to X-ray it *now* and then call me back. Is she in much pain?"

"Yes, but I didn't want to give her anything until I cleared it with an obstetrician."

"Well?"

"Well, he hasn't called back."

I am furious. "Let me speak to my son-in-law."

I explain to Dick what I think needs to be done. I tell him I'll call an orthopedic surgeon friend of mine in Chicago and ask if he can see Ann in consultation.

My friend agrees to see her. The X ray reveals a dislocated hip, not a fracture. Ann is moved by ambulance to Skokie Valley Hospital, where my friend is chief of orthopedic surgery. Her dislocated hip is reduced within two hours of making the diagnosis, but seven hours after the accident.

Whether the delay because of improper management at Resurrection Hospital will result in any permanent damage to her hip, we will know in time. Ann still has constant pain in her hip. Six months after the accident, she had to have a Caesarean section to deliver our first grandchild. But the baby is beautiful and completely healthy.

Although I was 2,000 miles away, I was able to act as my daughter's patient advocate and avoid more serious complications. I was also able to save Resurrection Hospital, its ER physician, and the orthopedic surgeon who refused to get out of bed from a malpractice suit based on their obvious negligence. However, my daughter was the only one who thanked me. ɜ☙

Another word of caution in dealing with the Medical Establishment concerns prescription drugs.

Drugs can be prescribed by their generic or chemical name, or by the brand name of the manufacturer, for example, ampicillin, a synthetic penicillin, is known by at least three different brand names: Amcill (manufactured by Parke-Davis), Omnipen (by Wyeth), and Principen (by Squibb). Most states have recently passed laws that permit a pharmacist to substitute the generic equivalent of a drug your physician has prescribed. This move was mostly a political football, designed to save money in government-reimbursed medical programs. Generic drugs are usually cheaper because they are not protected by trademark.

Pharmacists like the freedom to substitute generic equivalents because it allows them to stock only one brand, which is less expensive than carrying three or more. The cost of the specific brand you receive with a generic prescription will vary with the pharmacy. Chances are, if you call three different pharmacies and ask the price of a drug by its generic name, you will find three different prices. In other words, you will not necessarily save with the generic substitution program.

Moreover, generic equivalency is not necessarily the same as biological equivalency. Although the drug is the same in chemical composition, it may produce a different biological and therapeutic response when it is used in different physical forms. Such physical characteristics as particle size can affect the solubility and absorption of a drug. Different coatings on the tablets or capsules may cause the drug to be released in the intestinal tract in different ways. There is no standardization from manufacturer to manufacturer. Iron as ferrous sulfate, for instance, varies in solubility to the point where some preparations pass untouched through the intestinal tract.

Insulin is one drug that is notorious for the variation in its biological effect depending on the manufacturer. A few years ago, a group of diabetic patients who were well stabilized on a specific dose of insulin in the hospital went into insulin shock as soon as they went home. The patients were blamed for not following orders, until someone realized that the outpatient pharmacy was giving them insulin from a different manufacturer. The same dosage had a totally different biological effect.

So what can you, the consumer, do? You should insist that if your pharmacist is making a generic substitution in filling your prescription, the generic equivalent has also been shown to have biological equivalency. If your pharmacist can't assure you of this, don't accept the substitute, even though it is less expensive.

And what happens at the end? At the end comes death. Yet death is not the enemy. Disease is the enemy.

This confusion about what we are fighting, as perceived by many physicians, is not in the best interests of our patients. We lose sight of our goals, we flail in desperation at windmills, we continue to fight blindly after the final whistle has blown.

When death is assumed to be the enemy, the patient is frequently the victim. The senile old lady is transported across town three times a week to be dialyzed. The incurable cancer patient's final days are made miserable with chemotherapy because some researcher has reported: "The responders to this experimental drug lived longer than nonresponders." What a cruel hoax—of course they did, they were the biologically stronger of the group. But did the group as a whole, the responders and the nonresponders, live any longer than those that did not receive the drug? Probably not. And I doubt the misery of those extra one or two months was worth it.

When death is declared the enemy, the patient is maintained on life-support systems long after an EEG (electroencephalogram) shows brain death.

When disease is seen as the enemy, we try no less to cure the patient. Faced with a life-threatening condition, we take heroic measures in our attempt to save the patient's life. But the quality of the life extension we can offer becomes a factor in determining the extent to which we push heroics.

Lewis Thomas, writing in the *Wilson Quarterly*, speaks to the difference: "I do not believe there are any barriers to prevent our reaching a deep understanding of disease processes, and I see no reason why we should not be able ultimately to gain a reasonably satisfactory control over human disease in general. [On the other hand:] This has nothing to do with mortality. We will still die on schedule and probably on something pretty much like today's schedule, but I think we can spare ourselves the incapacitating and painful ailments that now make aging itself a sort of disease."*

Many physicians in their younger years—and I include myself—take the death of a patient as a personal failure. Some psychologically cut off their hands, as might have been literally done for them in ancient Egypt. A few do not recover; their confidence destroyed, they never achieve their optimal competency.

This overreaction to death has spread beyond the physician; it touches most health workers. In many of our hospitals it is impossible to die without an attempt at cardiopulmonary resuscitation, even for the terminally ill. The question is: Should there be a limit to these attempts? In most hospitals it takes a physician's signed order to omit CPR. And this is probably where the responsibility should rest, so that the patient with true accidental cardiac arrest, who can be resuscitated, will not be overlooked. Another possibility is to honor a "living will," a document signed when the patient is competent, which requests that no heroic measures be taken to prolong life. Still, the decision to let a patient die is an awesome one. I'll never forget one woman's reaction to my attempt to postpone her mother's death.

&§ Katherine is sitting in a chair in her mother's hospital room. Yesterday I operated and placed a pin in the old lady's broken hip.

* Lewis Thomas, Untitled.

Although she is in her eighties and somewhat senile, everything seems to be going well. Just this morning, I helped her dangle her legs on the side of the bed. But now she simply closes her eyes and dies.

I pull out all the stops. The words "code blue" to the operator summon droves of nurses and doctors and the CPR crash cart to the room. Katherine sits calmly in her chair throughout our frantic and unsuccessful attempt at resuscitation.

"I'm sorry," I finally said. "There was nothing we could do."

"I know," she replies. "Thank you. Now I would like to be alone with her for a few moments."

She is very gracious, but I will always remember the fleeting look of disdain I glimpse in her eyes. ❧

I believe we physicians have come to feel that death is the enemy because of the reactions of our patients' families to death. Few are as stoic as Katherine was. Breaking the news of a death is the physician's most difficult task. If this is also accompanied by a sense of failure, it is understandable that a doctor tries to forestall the inevitable.

On the other hand, I shall never forget my own mother's pleading to die in the terminal stages of metastatic cancer. Talking was difficult for her, but she forced out the words—her last—"Please, Tom; I want to die."

"I know, dear," was all I could say. If I could ever have believed in euthanasia, it was at that moment. What I did do was to make sure she slept through those final hours free of pain. And I thanked God when her tortured breathing stopped.

Can you imagine the horror of not being allowed to die?

All of us are taught to fear death. It is shrouded in mystery, talked of in hushed tones. We learn that the greatest crime is to cause the death of another. The ultimate expression of love is to die to save another's life. We rarely contemplate death directly, especially our own. Instead, we speculate on God and immortality. How we eventually face our own mortality is determined by our religious beliefs.

As a child, I was terrorized by my parents' fundamentalist religion with its hellfire and damnation. I rejected their faith and turned to my own brand of religious existentialism; it has served me well as a way of life. But it was only four years ago, as I prepared myself for major surgery, that I finally faced my own mortality and overcame the fear.

As I ponder on these experiences, I become convinced that it is only through the process of facing our own mortality that we attain maturity. Only then can we face the certainty of our own death with equanimity and become free to live. We also gain the inner resources necessary to help others with understanding and support.

It is at the end when the battle with disease has been lost, when death is inevitable, that we most need the services of a mature patient advocate in dealing with the Medical Establishment.

CHAPTER 20

Changing the American Way
of Medicine

CHANGING any entrenched system is difficult. The status quo is always the most comfortable. To tamper with it, people must perceive a marked advantage for themselves in a new situation, or they must see their present position as untenable. And usually it is necessary to have a realistic goal in sight before one becomes willing to move. People hate to walk in the dark, not knowing where the path is leading.

Perhaps this is why government has been so unsuccessful in its attempts to mold the American health care system. There has been no consensus on a national health policy; no one has painted a picture of a utopian system. And government has lost its credibility as a competent guide along an uncharted path.

Health care has been tossed about as a political football in America for the past twenty years. With nearly every election, a health care crisis was brought out of the closet to be used by some bright young men in Washington to forward their own careers. Everyone knew we had the best medical care system in the world, so it wouldn't do any harm to toss it around a bit, and it might be possible to score a few brownie points in the process.

There have been two halves in the game so far. The first half was nearly all offense. In the second half, the defense took over. The result was a stalemate, and we have gone into overtime.

The first half was played in the 1960s, and the offense was spectacular. There were breaks through the line on nearly every play. The medical team could do no wrong. The spectators went wild. They wanted the ball advanced to everyone. The goal was national health insurance. But every time they neared the goal line, they were stopped just short of the mark.

The second half was all defense; it was played in the 1970s. The game had gotten too big and it was costing too much. Every conceivable defensive strategy was tried, but it was difficult to control the advance. Toward the end of the half the political football had become a hot potato and nobody wanted to handle the ball. So it ended in stalemate.

What will happen in the 1980s is anyone's guess. So far, no one has scored, and the cost keeps going up.

There are still some bright young people in Washington who enjoy playing the game, although they don't seem to have quite as much enthusiasm as they had in the past. Most of them are on the staff of senators and representatives or the various congressional committees. Many have been in Washington for years; they seem to form a perpetual cadre that changes very little with elections or new administrations. Many resemble the bureaucracy they work in—unchanging, unresponsive, and unaccountable to the electorate. And it is these staff people who usually write the health legislation. Lobbyists talk to them more than to their bosses. They are the ones who know what is really going on. They have the power to control the direction of health care. And once their ideas become law, they simply pass the ball to other bright young staffers in the Department of Health and Human Services, who write the regulations necessary to implement the law. On occasion, regulations have been known to change the law to the point where it no longer reflects the intent of Congress.

Some of these enterprising staffers even have M.D. degrees. But they rarely reflect the thinking of the profession. Most joined the cadre directly after medical school or their residency. Very few have actually practiced medicine and most have never been sick.

It would be foolish to surrender the future direction of medical care in the United States to these bright young people, no matter how well intentioned they may be. Certainly their track record or that of government at any level does not warrant such trust. Their attempt to regulate the system during the past ten years through legislation has been a complete failure. The ill-conceived and poorly planned expansion of the system during the 1960s, especially the uncontrolled importation of foreign medical graduates, has resulted in a medical care system that is out of proportion with and totally unrelated to the real health and medical care needs of our nation. It is easy, therefore, to become disenchanted with government's impact on our system.

The games that were played with the medical care system over the past two decades have been a major factor in turning invented crises into the real dilemma we face today—runaway costs.

Now, we are told by the government, we have only two choices if we want to contain costs. We can have more of the same government interference, with increased attempts to regulate the system, approaching a public utility type of control. Or, we can create a competitive environment, in which knowledgeable consumers and providers make cost-effective choices, thus restoring market incentives as a control on the system. Unfortunately, the latter choice—Alain Enthoven's Consumer Choice Health Plan or its Republican offspring, described in Chapter 12—requires a radical reorganization of the present delivery system in order to be effective.

What we are faced with is a true dilemma—two equally unsatisfactory alternatives.

Certainly, regulation of the system over the past ten years has not reduced costs. Hospital costs, in particular, have continued to rise at an average annual rate of one and one-half times the Consumer Price Index, and in 1982 it was three times the CPI rate. Admittedly, Professional Standard Review Organizations have reduced Medicare expenditures chiefly by decreasing the length of stay. But this does not mean hospital costs are any lower. It is simply that the federal government's share in paying for them has been reduced. Payment has shifted to the other users of the hospital; in other words, the rest of us pay more.

Certificate-of-need legislation, restricting expansion, might have been a good idea. But it came too late to prevent the wasteful duplication of services and facilities in our system. An oversupply of expensive technology had already been created by fifty years of open-ended cost reimbursement of hospitals.

Prospective rate-setting commissions have cut hospital costs but have led to the bankruptcy of many hospitals. What happens is that the commission sets a per diem rate, which does not take into consideration the mix of patients with different diagnoses. It costs much more per day to care for a patient who is unconscious with a brain tumor than for a person convalescing from hepatitis. It also tends to cost more to care for the elderly and the poor because the illnesses that bring them to the hospital are generally severe and their overall health status may be low.

Hospitals in which a majority of the patients are covered by Medicare and Medicaid fare poorly under a system of set per diem rates. Usually these hospitals are in large urban areas, where they also serve the medically indigent (those not covered by Medicaid, yet too poor to pay for high-cost medical care) and illegal aliens (with no health insurance). Since Medicare and Medicaid will not share in the cost of payment for a hospital's bad debts, these costs must be shifted to the hospital's private patients. When a hospital has no private patients, it goes into bankruptcy. This usually occurs in areas with the greatest poverty and the greatest need for medical care. It is ironic that Medicare and Medicaid, programs designed to eliminate charity care for the elderly and the poor, are now increasing the need for charity and at the same time causing the demise of the charitable institutions, the public general and urban teaching hospitals, which in the past provided most of the free care.

After a decade of increasing frustration with regulation, most hospitals should welcome the relief offered by the competition strategy. After all, competition is not new to hospitals; they have been competing for doctors and patients for years. Every hospital has played the game of keeping up with the Joneses. If Jones's hospital put in a cobalt bomb, then Smith's hospital had to have one too, or its doctors would take all their patients needing cobalt treatment for cancer to Jones's hospital. Aided by the Hill-Burton Law (which provided the facilities) and cost reimbursement by Blue Cross and Medicare (which paid for new equipment), Smith had no trouble keeping up with or getting ahead of Jones. America ended up with the best-equipped hospitals in the world—and the cost of duplicated facilities and services. Is it not ironic, then, that competition, which added to health care costs, is now being offered as the way to bring them under control?

Enthoven's competition strategy, however, calls for regulated competition. Only players who meet certain standards and agree to abide by the rules will be allowed to play. Providers must reorganize into health maintenance organizations (HMOs) or other alternative setups. They have to contract with individuals on an annual basis for all their medical care. Consumers, in turn, are asked to sacrifice one of the basic tenets of American medicine—the right of free choice of a physician.

This proposal would drastically change the medical delivery system. It seems unlikely that either providers or consumers will willingly agree to it, even given the continued cost escalation. Both providers and consumers are generally satisfied with the present organization of our delivery system. Why should they give up the right to contract individually with a physician? Although physicians feel more strongly, both physicians and patients resent the intrusion of a third party into their contract, be it government or an insurance company. It is true that both have already become accustomed to third-party payment for medical care, and few would want to eliminate this from our system. But they want to keep the third party confined to that one aspect of the contract—payment for services rendered. They do not want the third party to dictate changes in the organization of the system and have a voice in determining what, how, when, and where services are provided.

I disagree with Enthoven and other advocates of competition strategies; we are not limited to two alternatives, regulation or competition. *There is a third path, one that incorporates the best aspects of the competition strategy and minimal regulation but does not require a reorganization of the delivery system or a sacrifice of the basic tenets of the American way of medicine.*

This third way is much more likely to succeed in controlling costs because it corrects the three primary causes of cost escalation: the financing mechanisms, the excess capacity of the system, and medicine's nearly exclusive preoccupation with the treatment of disease, to the neglect of prevention. Consumer choice and competition strategies ignore these other two important factors and concentrate on the financing mechanisms. Let me outline the advantages of this third alternative, point by point.

Controlling Hospital Costs

Enthoven's financial diagnosis of the malady in our system is correct. He has put his finger on the perverse incentives that are causing cost escalation. Cost reimbursement of hospitals is the most important one. If we could change this one element in our present system, the rest would eventually fall into line, although it might take longer than we can afford to wait.

Enthoven's prescribed therapy, however, doesn't deal with the problem of cost reimbursement directly. It depends on the acceptance of HMOs and capitation reimbursement by consumers and providers as preliminary first steps. The elimination of cost reimbursement of hospitals cannot be left to chance.

The most viable alternative to cost reimbursement is prospective rate-setting on a case rate basis, not a per diem one. In essence, this means we should establish, in advance, a fee schedule for hospital care based on a set charge for each diagnosis—just like the fee schedules Blue Shield has established for physicians' fees. For example, a patient with a principal diagnosis of acute appendicitis would receive a bill for a previously determined amount (the rate for acute appendicitis in that community), no matter how many tests were ordered, how much medication was given, how many complications developed, or how long the hospital stay was. Every purchaser of care—individuals, insurance companies, Blue Cross, Medicare, and Medicaid—would have to pay the same rate or fee.

The hospital, knowing it would receive only a set reimbursement for any patient with a particular diagnosis, would have a financial incentive to eliminate unnecessary tests and to keep the length of stay as short as possible. It would thus pressure its medical staff to behave in a cost-effective manner. There would be no need for utilization review or PSROs. In addition, this financial incentive would promote high-quality care because there would be an advantage in avoiding complications, which result in longer stays and higher costs. (Complications can usually be prevented by having medical care teams pay greater attention to detail.)

A prospective case rate system carries the same financial incentive to be cost-conscious as the capitation system of reimbursement. It can be thought of as capitation on a case-by-case basis. An example of how this works comes from the Illinois Masonic Medical Center in Chicago, where case rate data have been kept for the past ten years. For the last seven years, these data have been collected on the Hospital Utilization Program (HUP) discharge abstract, the data service used by this hospital. As medical director, I used these data to establish a profile of practice for each member of the medical staff. It was easy to identify physicians who, in treating the same disease, were consistently generating higher costs than their peers. Feedback of these data to the individual usually resulted in a change of behavior. Although this system was originally developed as a means of quality control, we soon learned that poor quality of care is usually associated with high cost. In other words, this method has an even greater potential for cost control.

New Jersey has been experimenting with prospective rate reimbursement using diagnostically related groups (DRGs) of diseases. A single rate is set for the entire group of diseases. For example, all diseases of the gallbladder are considered one group. The idea is that it is easier to set rates for a group than for each separate disease, although this seems unsophisticated given the specificity of medical record technology in our computer age. Certainly, the use of DRGs is less precise, a hospital can be reimbursed the same amount for a broken toe as for a broken leg in New Jersey. Still, although less acceptable, DRGs could be a viable alternative to case rate.

Whether one looks at a group of related diagnoses or only at cases with the same diagnosis, there will be a variation in the severity of the illness. Some cases will be hard to manage and others easy. On some, the hospital will make a profit; others will cost more than the case rate. But over a period of time these variations will balance each other. I believe, however, that the balance will be achieved more quickly and more equitably if the rate is based on individual diagnoses rather than on DRGs. (This balancing was certainly the experience of those of us who for years accepted Blue Shield rates as payment in full for our medical services.)

The important point is that prospective case rate reimbursement will have the same financial incentives to contain costs as the capitation method *without having to reorganize the delivery system.* Hospitals would not be required to become part of an HMO.

Legislation will be necessary to establish rate-setting commissions and mandate this method of payment, not only for federal programs but for all purchasers of care. The rate-setting commissions should probably be organized at the state level, but should establish various rates throughout a state to permit community rating. The federal government's role should be one of overseer, assuring equity in the system and monitoring federal programs.

Controlling Cost and Quality of Physicians' Services

Everyone should have a family doctor. The most appropriate physician for this role is the new specialist in family practice. In an ideal system, family practitioners would be primarily concerned with promoting the health of their patients and preventing disease. They would be the physisians of first contact for each episode of illness of their patients, with the knowledge and skills to personally treat 80% of those episodes. They would refer patients to appropriate specialists when and if they were needed. But after the need for this specialist ended, the patient would return to the family physician, who would be responsible for providing continuity of care over time. Ideally, in addition to the family practitioner the primary care team would include a patient educator, who would teach patients how to change their behavior to foster better health.

This type of primary care, in which health promotion and prevention of disease play significant parts, is not easily reimbursed on a traditional fee-for-service basis. It is much more compatible with a capitation reimbursement method because many doctor visits will not be for the treatment of illness, but for well-care. Therefore, capitation reimbursement should be offered as an alternative method of payment.

The same commission that determines the prospective case rates for hospital care should publish a guide for consumers, giving community-rated annual capitation fees for primary care. Capitation reimbursement would not be the mandated method of payment, although capitation fees should be set at a level at which family physicians would see this mode of payment, with its guaranteed annual income, as being equally advantageous to them as fee-for-service payment.

Consumers would then have a choice of capitation or fee-for-service payment for their primary care. Knowing the published capitation fee rate for their community, they would be in a position to judge which method of payment was to their advantage. They could make an effective choice in a competitive free market. Moreover, at any time they could switch from fee-for-service to capitation payment, with the understanding that they would be making a financial commitment to continue the capitation fee for one year.

The capitation method of payment for primary care has several advantages for consumers. First, the physician has a financial incentive to keep them well through active preventive medicine and health promotion services. Second, they are guaranteed a family doctor who will provide continuity of care. Third, they will have a patient advocate, someone who will be on their side in dealing with the medical maze. Fourth, the physician will have no financial incentive to overtreat or order unnecessary tests, since the physician will be expected to pay for *all* services he orders out of the capitation fee. Fifth, there is a financial incentive for the family physician to refer the patient to a specialist when it becomes necessary as no additional fees will be paid to the family doctor and payment for the specialist does not come out of the capitation fee. (This eliminates the current practice of some primary care physicians of holding on to the patient too long when they should be seeking consultations.)

Perhaps the greatest potential advantage for the consumer under the capitation method of payment for primary care will be the elimination of the current wide variation in cost when the same condition is treated by a family physician and an internal medicine specialist. Under capitation, the internist, in order to compete with the family physician in providing primary care, would have to charge the same capitation fee.

Several alternative organizational arrangements would be possible with capitation reimbursement for primary care. At the simplest level, the family practitioner could bill the patient directly for an annual capitation fee. In this situation, a contract could be signed, spelling out the expectations of both parties and determining in advance what services would be included in the agreement. (The rate-setting commission would also define the scope of services used in determining the capitation fee.)

At another level, several family physicians could form a primary care HMO, limited to family physicians and providing only primary care. Again, a contract could be made directly with prospective patients. This HMO could take the form of a prepaid group practice or an independent practice association (IPA) of family practitioners. Unlike a comprehensive care HMO, however, a primary care HMO would not need to provide specialist services, so that there would be less financial risk and greater ease of organization.

With a capitation system, health insurance companies could provide comprehensive coverage plans that would include primary care services. Under the fee-for-service system, it has proved actuarily unsound for insurance companies to include office visits or other primary care services in their policies. A fixed capitation fee, however, could easily be added to present hospitalization insurance. Health insurance companies could pay out the capitation fee to the patient's chosen provider, be it an individual practitioner, a group, or an HMO.

Of course, there would need to be checks on a capitation system to prevent abuse of the physician's time by unnecessary demands. For instance, the patient might be required to make some token out-of-pocket payment for each visit other than for routinely scheduled appointments for preventive and well-care.

I believe capitation reimbursement for primary care could become the preferred method for both patients and physicians if it is phased in slowly and voluntarily. The main advantage of this approach is its potential for making the appropriate changes in financial incentives *without requiring a reorganization of the delivery system.*

Specialists, when not providing primary care, could continue to be reimbursed on a fee-for-service basis. Pediatricians, for example, could provide their primary care services for an annual capitation fee. More specialized pediatricians, such as neonatologists and pediatric cardiologists, would charge on a fee-for-service basis. Similarly, obstetricians should be willing to contract for a fixed capitation fee for care of a pregnancy— which they claim is primary care—whether or not a complication develops that requires a Caesarean.

The point is that once the cost of primary care is contained by having a large portion of it reimbursed by the capitation method, the new system will add its own controls to those already existing to keep the fee-for-service reimbursement in line, not only at the primary care level but for secondary and tertiary care specialists as well.

With a family physician, consumers will acquire a patient advocate to guide them in choosing a specialist when necessary. Specialists would be competing for the family physician's referrals on the basis of the quality of their care and the fees they charge. In other words, the system would automatically exert controls over quality of care and appropriate fees. Another control would simply be the rate-setting commission's publication of customary fees for common procedures in each community. This list would serve as an effective guide for consumers. Also, since specialists' fees for procedures would still be insured under the present Blue Shield and commercial indemnity plans, they would continue to exert their own pressure in the form of fee schedules.

Indirectly, the academic medical centers would also benefit from this approach. In a strictly competitive environment, these institutions would have difficulty unless new mechanisms were established to pay for medical education. Yet they could function well under a system combining prospective case rates with continued fee-for-service reimbursement of specialists. The nature of tertiary care would command a larger fee and a higher case rate than that for secondary care given in community hospitals. The costs of education could be built into the case rate.

To facilitate the transfer of patients needing tertiary care, the academic medical centers should enlarge their affiliation agreements with community hospitals and with groups of physicians providing primary care in their service area. This would also extend the educational environment to the entire system. Physicians should be trained where patients are treated, not exclusively in the medical school or teaching hospital. With this type of arrangement, undergraduate, graduate, and continuing medical education could become a continuum throughout the professional life of a practicing physician, and the quality of care at all levels would improve.

Controlling the Excess Capacity of the System

Little attention has been paid to the excess capacity of our system as it exists today. But this factor is probably as important as the perverse financial incentives in causing cost escalation.

The Graduate Medical Education National Advisory Committee report, discussed in Chapter 13, clearly indicates this excess capacity. It predicts that by 1990 we will have a surplus of 70,000 physicians and, by 2000, an even more serious surplus of 120,000.

Remember that 80% of our physicians today are specialists, when the need is for 20%. Although the new family practitioners could handle 80% of the conditions for which patients consult a doctor, they number only 14% of practicing physicians. As a result, we often end up with a physician who is overqualified to care for our problem and who overtreats us, at a higher cost than necessary.

Most primary care today is provided by three specialists—internists, pediatricians, and obstetrician/gynecologists—instead of a single primary care practitioner. These specialists generally set their fees according to their board certification, not according to the service needed. In other words, their fees for primary care reflect the higher cost of their specialized training.

In addition to this overspecialization, a major cause of cost escalation is our love affair with technology, which in fact spawned the overspecialization. The tendency has been to use the most sophisticated equipment available, without regard for cost or need.

We have the best medical care system in the world; I am not questioning that. And we should retain our present capabilities in all the specialties. But we do not need the quantity of specialists and sophisticated machines we now support to do this. Unless the numbers change, we will continue to provide care that is more related to the profession's accomplishments than to the American people's needs.

Most physicians continue to act as if our resources were infinite, as if they had been given a blank check by the people. A dictum from government is not the answer to this situation, however; coercion from without rarely is. Leadership must come from within if we are to retain the autonomy and right of self-determination of the profession. Physicians must actively restructure the physician component of our medical care system to meet the needs of the American people.

The immediate need is a drastic change in the numbers and types of physicians we educate. The Accreditation Council on Graduate Medical Education already has the power to make these changes, if the profession concurs. We need to assure everyone access to a family physician. The ideal proportion would be 50% family practitioners, 17% specialists providing some primary care (*i.e.*, general internists, pediatricians, and obstetrician/gynecologists), and 33% specialists providing secondary and tertiary care. (These percentages are based on the findings of the Hunterdon System in Flemington, New Jersey, and the Kaiser Plan in northern California. In both settings, the ratio of generalists to specialists was controlled to provide the most cost-effective care of high quality. In both, the ideal ratio was two primary care physicians to one specialist.)

Paying Attention to Prevention

Closely related to our current problem of oversupply is our preoccupation with treating disease and our neglect of prevention. Most physicians seem unaware that we are in the midst of an epidemiological revolution. Infectious diseases have been brought under control, yet our system is organized as though we were still in the middle of this battle. What we face today is a new group of killers—the chronic diseases, with heart disease, cancer, and stroke in the lead. They will not succumb to the same line of attack.

Our approach to coronary heart disease emphasizes a highly expensive operation—coronary bypass surgery (remember Adam Americus's experience). Prevention is slighted. Yet Dr. John Fahrquar, director of the Stanford Heart Disease Prevention Program, believes we can prevent 90% of atherosclerotic heart disease and stroke simply by appropriate intervening to eliminate just three risk factors: cigarette smoking, high blood pressure, and elevated serum cholesterol. And this can be done through proven techniques for smoking cessation programs, combined with appropriate diet, exercise, and stress management, which can be provided at a fraction of the cost of coronary bypass surgery.

The same point can be made with lung cancer. At present we can cure only 10% of lung cancer. Yet we could prevent 90% of lung cancer simply by eliminating cigarette smoking. The bottom line is that *90% of the three leading causes of death in America—accounting for 70% of the total deaths—could be prevented by risk factor intervention.*

Moreover, 50% of *all* disease today could be prevented—a potential saving of over $100 billion per year. Unfortunately, we, as a profession, have not been willing to admit this, even to ourselves. We have not been willing to change our nearly total concern with the treatment of disease and give equal consideration to prevention and to promotion of health. Physicians are directly responsible for the fact that in 1981 Americans spent 96% of their health care dollars on treatment and only 4% on prevention and health promotion, out of a total of $287 billion.

A utopian system can never be realized, but we can achieve a better system, which will control costs and maintain quality. It is not beyond our reach. The Plan I have advocated keeps the best parts of our present system intact; no radical reorganization into HMOs or other configurations is required. Only three fundamental changes are necessary. Let me summarize:

1. We must change the financing mechanisms to remove the perverse incentives of our present system. We must change from open-ended cost reimbursement of hospitals to prospective case rates. We must offer an alternative to fee-for-service payment for primary care in the form of an annual community-rated capitation fee.

2. We must assure everyone access to a family physician by changing the numbers and types of physicians we educate to meet the proven cost-effective proportion of twice as many primary care physicians as specialists, with at least 50% family practitioners.

3. We must change our almost exclusive emphasis on treatment of disease to give equal consideration to prevention of disease and promotion of health.

Health promotion and wellness will be much easier to establish as an important element in the system once the first two changes are accomplished. The majority of physicians will be family practitioners, and they will have a financial incentive, as well as a professional motivation, to keep people well. Specialists, who must rightly emphasize the treatment of disease, will still be able to provide the best possible care, but without bankrupting us. No one wants to destroy the treatment capabilities of our specialists or to eliminate the advanced technology that supports them; we simply want to restore a rational balance that matches the system to the nation's health and medical care needs.

How close we can come to this utopian system will depend to a large degree on physicians. Will they be willing to disrupt the status quo enough to bring about these necessary changes? Can they be made to see the necessity for mutual coercion to protect the medical commons? Unless physicians take a leadership role in bringing us out of our present dilemma, the profession could easily lose its autonomy to the other forces in the Medical Establishment. And the quality of care might then be diminished if the physician becomes a captive of the hospitals, the health insurance industry, or the pharmaceutical manufacturers.

Robert Cunningham, an astute observer of our system, has expressed a similar concern in a recent issue of *Trustee*. Looking at the government's new competition strategies, which focus solely on cost control, he indicates that we may be moving from trying to deliver the highest quality care at the lowest possible price to delivering low-cost care at the highest possible quality—in other words shifting the priority from the quality of health care to its costs. If this occurs, we may witness the demise of America as the leader in medical care.

How can we prevent this from happening? Is it only up to the physicians? Or can you, as a consumer, also become a force for changing the system and making it respond to your health care needs? I believe you can—by taking the route described in the next part of this book.

PART TWO

How to Reclaim Your Own Life

CHAPTER 21

Prevention Is the Best Cure— and the Least Expensive

THE AMERICAN MALE is killing himself. Our mortality and morbidity rates for white adult males in each decade of life far exceed those of any other industrialized country. During the 1970s, for men aged forty-five to fifty-four, there were 9,306 deaths per million per year in the U.S., compared with 7,384 in Canada, 7,090 in England, 5,521 in Sweden, and 3,982 in the Netherlands.*

For American men aged fifteen to twenty-four, Suicide itself is the third leading cause of death. Even more, these young men are prone to knocking themselves (and others) off with motor vehicles—their leading cause of death. Since 50% of these accidents are associated with drunken driving, they may well represent another mode of suicide.

By the time the American male has reached the mature age of forty-five to sixty-four, he has developed many more sophisticated and subtle ways of doing himself in. Clear-cut, intentional suicide is less frequent. Most of us have learned how to keep passing the open window, perhaps because the finality of the act is clearer. In any case, using the police definition, suicide drops to sixth in the ten leading causes of death in this age group, and motor vehicle accidents to seventh.

But there are other, equally sure ways of killing yourself. Most of these go undetected. They blend in with our modern lifestyle so well that no one notices who in the crowd is on the road to suicide. These "in" methods may be slower, but they are no less deadly. The best part is that there is no way you can change your mind at the last minute. The cumu-

* Statistics are available at this time only for the American male. Women, however, have entered the work force in greater numbers in the past decade and have been subjected to the same environmental stresses. It is inconceivable that they will not soon be experiencing the same increased morbidity and mortality as their male counterparts. But because women have a premenopausal hormonal protection against coronary heart disease, they have been excluded from some epidemiologic studies that include this cause of morbidity and mortality for those under fifty years of age. (However, see a further discussion of these male and female differences in Chapter 24.)

lative effect will get you. One small dose of a killer may be relatively harmless, but taken over twenty years or more it is poison.

Cigarette smoking is the most popular method. It is used by 50 million Americans. I was one of them. Of course, I never thought of cigarette smoking as a form of suicide. And that's the sad part; most of the 50 million won't realize it until it is too late.

~§ I started smoking at age eighteen. I was a sophomore in college, and the most important thing in my life was to be accepted by my peers. Anyone who was anyone smoked. It took me two years to learn how to inhale. That was 1938. By the time World War II rolled around and Lucky Strike green went to war, I was hooked. I resorted to Bull Durham and rolled my own. After I entered the service, I could get all the cigarettes I wanted at the PX for half the civilian price. I smoked up a storm.

I was one of the 105,000 physicians who did not stop smoking when the Surgeon General's first report on smoking was issued in 1964. Smoking may be hazardous to your health, I agreed. But not to the point where I felt I should quit. My only acquiescence was to switch to low-tar filtered cigarettes. I started with Kents but as soon as a lower tar content cigarette was placed on the market, I switched. The last ten years I smoked only Carlton, the lowest—but I was smoking about three packs a day to compensate.

I rationalized my habit in the usual ways, using the standard clichés. I would intone Madison Avenue, repeating their pitch about low-tar cigarettes every time I lit one. I would tell myself that no one in my family had ever had lung cancer. (I persisted in this one even after an uncle died of lung cancer in the late 1960s; an uncle seemed too far removed to affect my genes.)

My favorite line was: "By the time I get my lung cancer, they will have developed a cure." I felt very loyal to my profession when I used this. And, of course, my ego chimed in: "It may happen to others but it won't happen to me. After all, I'm a physician; we cure diseases, we don't get them."

But it did happen to me. And they hadn't yet found the cure.

Ironically, the first symptoms of my cancer began the day I quit smoking, on February 21, 1978. About a year before I had been invited by the late John Knowles, then president of the Rockefeller Foundation, to attend a workshop in New York on future directions of U.S. health policy. In addition to the Rockefeller Foundation, the workshop was cosponsored by the Blue Cross Association, the Institute of Medicine of the National Academy of Sciences, and the Health Policy Program of the University of California, San Francisco. They had assembled an impressive list of authorities. From the evidence they presented, I left that workshop convinced that prevention would be the key factor in America's future health care policy.

After much study and further investigation, I decided to form a company to market health promotion and preventive medicine services. The workplace would be our target.

But I soon realized that I had to be my own first client. I couldn't sell health promotion if I smoked. I enrolled in SmokEnders, a commercial smoking cessation program, and successfuly quit smoking five weeks later, on February 21, 1978.

It was that day that I began to cough, and I continued to cough for a whole year. I hate to admit it, but despite the fact that I am a physician, and even though I had access to the best medical care throughout that year, it took until February 23, 1979, to find the cause of my cough. Hidden behind my heart was a cancer of the lung that did not show up on routine chest X rays. Only when they did tomograms—special X rays that take serial views of tissue slices, one centimeter apart—was the tumor found.

The next day I headed for M.D. Anderson Hospital and Tumor Institute in Houston, Texas, one of the country's best-known cancer centers. The rest of the story I have recounted in other parts of this book. I was lucky, or God had plans I didn't know about. I had an excellent surgeon, who removed my left lung and the contained cancer. This was followed by immunochemotherapy. I was rescued, and now I am in the process of reclaiming my own life.

I was unintentionally committing suicide. When I realized what I was doing, it was almost too late.

The other 50 million smokers may not be as lucky as I was. In 1979, the Surgeon General removed the "may be" from his warning: "Smoking is dangerous to your health." There is absolutely no question that 90% of cancer of the lung is caused by cigarette smoking. And although we are not sure of the mechanism, there is also no doubt that cigarette smoking plays a major role in causing atherosclerotic heart disease, the leading cause of death.

Cigarette smoking is used thirty-five times more often than all of the obvious means combined that individuals use to commit suicide, including firearms, razors, hanging, overdosing with drugs, jumping, drowning, or leaping in front of trains and trucks, and asps.

But smoking is not the only hidden method of suicide. Alcohol, faulty nutrition, overuse of medication, fast driving, and stress caused by the pressure to achieve are others, often found in combination, for a more certain effect. These personal behaviors are the major factors for both sexes in seven out of the ten leading causes of death in the U.S. today for those forty-five to sixty-four.

The leading causes of death vary with age groups and sex. In both sexes, however, for infants under one year, developmental problems associated with prematurity at birth are the number one killer. From one to fourteen years, the leading cause of death is some type of accident, with almost half associated with motor vehicles. Young adults, aged fifteen to twenty-four, usually die traumatic deaths—from motor vehicles, other accidents, suicide, or homicide, in that order.

For adults aged twenty-five to forty-four, cancer is the big killer, followed by heart disease, motor vehicle and other accidents, suicide and homicide, cirrhosis of the liver, stroke, influenza and pneumonia, and diabetes. Seventy percent of all adults who die between age forty-five and sixty-four die of the big three: heart disease, cancer, or stroke. For those over sixty-five, heart disease remains number one, followed by cancer, stroke, influenza and pneumonia, arteriosclerosis, diabetes, accidents, other respiratory diseases, cirrhosis, and motor vehicle accidents.

For our total population, all ages, both sexes, the ten leading causes of death are: (1) heart disease, (2) cancer, (3) stroke, (4) accidents other than motor vehicle accidents, (5) influenza and pneumonia, (6) motor vehicle accidents, (7) diabetes, (8) cirrhosis, (9) suicide, and (10) arteriosclerosis.

Experts at the Centers for Disease Control, a government agency that collects all the morbidity and mortality data throughout the country on a weekly basis, analyzed these ten leading causes of death in an attempt to identify the basic contributing factors for each condition or disease. They discovered that 50% of U.S. mortality (and morbidity) is due to unhealthy behavior or lifestyle, 20% to environmental hazards, 20% to human biological factors (including heredity), and 10% to inadequacies in the existing health care system.

This would seem to indicate that improving our medical care system would affect only 10% of the leading causes of mortality. We must, therefore, give most of our attention to these other factors in order to have an impact on the major causes of death and disability, especially behavioral and environmental factors.

Viewed from the opposite perspective, this means that the existing Medical Establishment, because it has little interest in prevention in general, and does not try to change patients' unhealthy behavior and life-style in particular, will have no effect on the elimination of 90% of the diseases that are causing most disability and death today. We, the people, are caught in the middle. The Medical Establishment keeps firing its cannons over our heads to remind us that we probably will need them sometime in our lives. And, it is true, we want to keep some of them there. But we can no longer afford all those different guns and all the technicians to run them. There are too many of them; more than we will ever need. "But we are busy," they cry. "How can you say there are too many of us?"

"Because you are treating, not curing, chronic diseases that could be prevented in the first place," we respond.

"How can you prevent a disease when you don't know its cause or cure?"

"It is not necessary to understand the cause or find a cure if effective preventive measures are available. Smallpox is a good example. We recently wiped smallpox off the face of the earth. Since 1796, this viral infection, once one of our most dreaded plagues, has been successfully curtailed by Edward Jenner's innoculation with cowpox matter. Jenner did not know the cause of smallpox, nor did he have a cure. He didn't even understand the nature of active immunity. It was 115 years before the cause of smallpox, a virus, was discovered in 1915. Now we've eradicated the disease, even though we never did find a cure."

"Jenner was just lucky. That's certainly not the scientific approach. Our technology will find the answers. Most people are still happy with what we are doing. So let's keep it that way. You do your thing; we'll do ours."

And that is the standoff we, the people, are caught in. The Medical Establishment is satisfied with the status quo. Experts have told us that today 50% of all disease is preventable, but the Medical Establishment isn't interested. Its concern is treatment, not prevention or the promotion of health. Medical costs, especially hospital costs, keep rising faster than the Consumer Price Index. And since the government is the largest purchaser of medical care, these costs are inflating the federal budget. The Medical Establishment grows richer, and we are approaching bankruptcy.

Everything points to the need for change in our system. So why does the Medical Establishment resist any move away from the status quo? We know there is a financial incentive for us to be sick, and we know that physicians are really only interested in the sick individual, but why is this most noble of all professions selling out to the financial interests of the rest of the Medical Establishment? Are physicians captives of the system? Are we witnessing the final desecration of the Hippocratic Oath? Or has there been a battle on Mount Olympus, with us, the mere mortals, left to suffer the consequences? Has Panacea usurped all the powers of her father, Aschlepius, and thrown out her sister Hygeia, who is concerned with living wisely and preserving health, so that she wanders aimlessly outside the realm of Medicine? It would be so easy if we could blame the gods.

There are those who advocate a totally new system of health promotion and prevention outside the practice of medicine, leaving treatment as the forte of the physician. The vendors at the flea market of health alternatives hope this will happen, although they would like a piece of the action in treatment as well. In California, chiropractors are beginning to fill the vacuum left by the absence of physician interest in health promotion. They have asked to have California law changed to include nutritional counseling as part of the practice of chiropractic work.

Polarity therapy, naturopathy, acupuncture, massage, yoga, EST, transcendental meditation, transactional analysis, nutritional counseling, food fads, even fortune telling—the list is a mile long. All claim to have the answers the public can't get from the medical profession.

This, I believe, is the real danger of medicine's reluctance to become involved in helping people stay healthy—it is impossible to tell what is good and what is harmful in that flea market. There is meaningless licensure, no regulation, and no quality control. However loving and well-meaning they are, some of the zealots out there could be more dangerous than the faith healers of a century ago.

We must insist that the practice of medicine not be confined to the diagnosis and treatment of disease or injury but include the preservation and restoration of health.

The American people have already moved to a position of marked interest in health promotion. Beginning in the mid-1960s, on their own, many turned to healthier lifestyles. Jogging became a national pastime, health food stores mushroomed, we switched from high-cholesterol animal fats to cholesterol-free vegetable fats. Soon, there was a striking decrease in deaths from coronary heart disease—a 22% decline from 1968 to 1977. This drop also coincided with a decrease in cigarette smoking by men and a marked increase in the number of men with high blood pressure who underwent treatment. In Europe during this same period there was no change in the mortality rate from heart disease, nor was there a decrease in such risk factors as smoking, hypertension, high cholesterol, and lack of exercise.

Cause and effect? Most investigators believe so. They also point to the increase in lung cancer in women. With a twenty-year gap to allow for the effect over time, this rise parallels the increase in cigarette smoking by women. As women are leaving the relative safety of the home and gaining equality with men in most areas of life, their health hazards are beginning to be the same as for men. We should anticipate less difference in the health status of the sexes. For example, it is thought that by 1983 lung cancer (the most common cancer in men) will replace breast cancer as the most common cancer in women. In seeking equality, women may not have anticipated the added risks of adopting men's lifestyles.

But there is good news. To prevent at least 50% of disease we need to change only a few unhealthy behaviors and lifestyles. We might save $120 billion in health care expenditures. But even more important, most of us can lead healthier and happier lives. All we have to do is convince the Medical Establishment.

And we, the people, might just be able to do that—if enough of us take the matter into our own hands. Look at what happened with the American automobile industry. Like the Medical Establishment, it became a victim of its own technology, blinded by the dazzle of the great god Technos. American cars kept getting bigger, with more automation, greater horsepower, more cylinders, more chrome. And they used more gas. They became ludicrous in a world of gas shortages, crowded highways, fewer parking spaces. So Detroit, the pride of industrial America, became bankrupt. Why? Because consumers stopped buying its product.

The consumers of health care can do the same. We can force the Medical Establishment to change, make it conform to our health care needs, by not buying its present produce. We can reclaim our own lives from the Medical Establishment. And there is a bonus—by taking responsibility for our own health, we will become more healthy in the process. If we can prevent 50% of illness through our own efforts, we will bring enough leverage to bear on the Medical Establishment to change its orientation to one that gives equal consideration to health promotion, wellness, and prevention of disease. Those who are well will learn how to stay well and those who have been less well will learn how to reach a higher level of wellness and stay there.

CHAPTER 22

Medicine's New
Crystal Ball

Now you can have your medical fortune told. No, medicine has not reverted to sorcery. It has entered the age of cybernetics. The computer has made it possible to analyze medical data with the aid of the mathematics of epidemiology and biostatistics. Using data compiled by the health insurance industry for actuarial purposes, this new technology allows us to examine any disease process to identify the *risk factors* that increase the probability of developing that specific disease.

It is also possible to analyze an individual's medical, family, and social history, and especially his or her lifestyle, to identify these same risk factors. The computer can then weigh the significance of the risk factors and determine whether or not, and to what degree, they constitute a hazard to the individual's health.

Health hazards can be identified in advance—years before they might show up on a routine physical examination or cause symptoms. They can be identified early enough to enable individuals to change those elements in their life that are creating the risk. And by making these changes, people can prevent disease.

For example, an analysis of coronary heart disease shows that you have a greater risk of developing a coronary if you are male, have a family history of the disease, are over fifty, overweight, smoke, get little exercise, have a stressful job, have high blood pressure and high blood levels of cholesterol, triglycerides, and low-density lipoproteins. There is nothing you can do about being male, over fifty, or having a family history of heart disease. But you can do a lot about the other risk factors. Many can be eliminated by changing your lifestyle.

Risk factors fall into three main categories: biological, environmental, and behavioral.

Biological factors are inherited. For some illnesses, like sickle-cell anemia and hemophilia, the inherited factors are specific and definite. With others, such as heart disease, diabetes, and some cancers, there is only a biological susceptibility to the diseases. Usually, however, the biological factors are strongly influenced by environment and behavior. For example, Japanese people who move to the United States tend to acquire in a few years the cancer risks of Americans rather than those of Japanese people who remain in Japan.

Environmental factors that contribute to disease have traditionally been the province of our public health system. Control of these factors has been accomplished by the collective action of society, usually by governmental agencies, using legal sanctions when necessary. Little is perceived to be under the control of the individual.

In this century, our public health system has improved our health environment by purifying our drinking water, disposing of sewage, pastuerizing milk and dairy products and enforcing other sanitary controls on our food supply, isolating and quarantining infectious individuals and animals, and conducting mass immunization programs.

In recent decades, however, as one hazard to our health is removed, several new potential hazards pop up. About a thousand new synthetic chemicals are developed each year. The aerial spraying of pesticides, the smokestacks and liquid wastes of manufacturing plants, the exhaust of the internal combustion engine, nuclear fallout, aerosols transporting hair spray and underarm deodorant, all pollute our air and water supply. We do not know the long-term effects of these contaminants referred to by scientists as *xenobiotics*—any foreign substance that has an effect on our biological systems.

Many biological and environmental risk factors can be intensified by unhealthy behaviors. This is especially true for uranium miners and asbestos workers. The combination of exposure to asbestos and smoking has a synergistic effect, intensifying these risk factors; their danger is far greater together than alone. Asbestos workers who smoke are thirty times more likely to develop lung cancer than asbestos workers who do not smoke, and ninety times more likely than an individual who neither smokes nor is exposed to asbestos.

But asbestos exposure is also dangerous for nonsmokers. A friend of a doctor friend of mine in New Jersey recently died of a mesothelioma, a specific type of lung cancer associated with inhaling asbestos fibers, twenty years after working for a single summer vacation in an asbestos plant. Those of you who have artificial gas fireplaces should make sure the "embers" that glow under your artificial logs are not asbestos—many are. A down-draft could destroy the relative safety of your hearth.

A supportive environment is also necessary for the health of most of us. The family plays an enormous role in protecting us from emotional hazards. Conversely, there is frequently a prodromal event, such as the death of a loved one, a divorce, the loss of a job, or simply the loss of a supportive environment, that triggers a serious illness. In a recent study into why people chose a particular time to seek medical attention at an emergency room, it was found that most had had the condition that made them seek help for some time. But it was a recent emotional upset that exacerbated the condition and precipitated the emergency visit.

Certain environmental risk factors are rarely under the control of the individual, and these include socioeconomic conditions. Poverty, poor housing, unemployment, and lack of education can result in inadequate nutrition, lack of preventive health services, frustration, and stress. It is these socioeconomic risk factors rather than biological ones that are responsible for higher mortality and morbidity in our nonwhite citizens.

It is the behavioral risk factors that are the most amenable to change, and it is change in this area that has the greatest potential for improving our health status. The remaining chapters of this book will focus on the means of identifying and eliminating these behavioral risks. As we saw in the last chapter, 50% of the deaths from the ten leading causes can be attributed to an unhealthy lifestyle.

The risk factors for the three leading causes of death and disability—heart disease, cancer, and stroke—are all very similar. Since these three diseases constitute 70% of our present-day mortality, eliminating relatively few risk factors in our lifestyle will pay large dividends.

The idea of risk factor intervention was first introduced to the medical profession in 1970, when Lewis Robbins and Jack Hall published their treatise *How to Practice Prospective Medicine*. They used a computerized system of matching behavioral risk factors with an individual's lifestyle, a method that Robbins had developed as a medical officer in the Public Health Service. They called their new tool a Health Hazard Appraisal (HHA). Physicians could identify for their patients the risk factors with a high probability of causing disease in the next five or ten years—hence, the title *Prospective Medicine*.

Robbins and Hall anticipated that their method would be used by the new family practitioners as part of the periodic health evaluations used in the continuing care of their patients. Yet, except for these new family practice specialists and the 300 physicians who belong to the Society of Prospective Medicine, the medical profession has generally ignored this breakthrough in the field of preventive medicine—for reasons that should now be obvious to the reader of this book.

Prospective medicine separates the risk factors for each disease into sex, race, and five-year age groups. As we have seen, each group has its special hazards. For example, the main health hazard for a sixteen-year-old white male is the key to his father's car. Unfortunately, the main health hazard for a sixteen-year-old black male is his own switchblade.

These behavioral risk factors—the ones we can do something about—are sometimes referred to as determinants of health. In an HHA, each determinant is weighted for its significance as a hazard to our health. One determinant may be a risk factor for several diseases. Cigarette smoking, for instance, is an important risk factor in lung cancer, heart disease, stroke, bronchitis, and emphysema.

To complete an HHA, the person fills out a simple questionnaire on his or her lifestyle; a computer then processes this information, and the computer printout is fed back to the individual. More sophisticated determinations of risk factors are possible, if one adds prognostically significant physical measurements, such as height and weight, blood pressure, and levels of blood sugar, cholesterol, triglycerides, and low- and high-density lipoproteins.

As we shall see, the HHA is not an end in itself; it is a motivational tool in prospective medicine's approach to disease prevention. And disease prevention is not an end in itself; it is just a first step in achieving a high level of wellness in body, mind, and spirit, which is the true definition of a healthy individual—much more than the mere absence of disease.

In the ten years that prospective medicine has been practiced, the HHA has been acknowledged as its key to success. The results of the HHA have provided the motivation necessary to overcome the malaise and inertia that makes any change difficult, especially one requiring a modification of behavior. Most health propaganda has no effect on the individual. Quoting mortality rates or some other statistics has little meaning. It's always the other guy, not me, they are referring to. We don't read the Surgeon General's warning on the Marlboro billboard ad; all we see is the macho cowboy lighting up in the saddle in the sunset.

But the HHA printout, that's different. That's *me* they're talking about; that's *my* life expectancy. I can add ten years to *my* life if *I* stop smoking. That's motivation; or, as I prefer, enlightened self-interest.

CHAPTER 23

How to Identify Your Own Health Hazards: Taking the First Step on the Road to Wellness

PROMOTING health and preventing disease are part of the same process. In the days when we were faced with a high incidence of infectious diseases, prevention was easy to understand. The physician was responsible for immunizing individuals and the public health system took care of sanitation in the handling of food and water. Little was required of the individual.

Today, however, we are dealing with the chronic diseases, half of which are caused by unhealthy behavior and lifestyles. The responsibility of the individual is clearer. Yet most individuals are not aware of the specific hazards to their health. And even if they are aware of a hazard, it's usually not in terms that carry personal meaning.

As we saw in the last chapter, medical science, with the help of the computer, can now analyze an individual's lifestyle and feed back the results in terms that will probably be significant to the individual—in terms of remaining years of life expectancy. When people learn that a particular habit is decreasing their own life expectancy by so many years, that usually gets their attention. You don't have to hit a forty-five-year-old man on the head with a two-by-four if he reads that he has less than ten more years to live if he continues with his present lifestyle.

This awareness is a necessary first step in changing behavior. And that is why the Health Hazard Appraisal is such an important assessment tool.

Most computer printouts of an HHA provided individuals with a score in terms of an appraisal age that they can compare with their actual age. For example, a fifty-five-year-old white female whose biological, environmental, and behavioral risk factors are all favorable might have an appraisal age of forty-five; this means she has a life expectancy that is ten years longer than the average for her peer group. Another fifty-five-year-old white female whose biological and environmental risk factors are equally favorable, but who leads a very unhealthy lifestyle, might have an appraisal age of sixty-five, with a life expectancy of ten years less than the average person in her peer group.

This same woman, however, would also be given an achievable age score. For example, she might be told she could achieve the same risk as an individual aged fifty—five years, younger than her actual age—if she changed specific behaviors for each of several risk factors. In other words, she could add fifteen years to her present life expectancy by appropriate behavioral change.

"But," you may say, "I don't have to bother with all this computer gadgetry. My doctor gives me an annual physical examination. It might cost more, but won't I get the same information?"

Unfortunately, no. Ideally, your physician would use an HHA as part of your periodic health evaluations (notice I did not say annual physical). But no, an annual physical cannot provide this same information. You are correct on one thing, however: The physical could cost you about twenty times more than an HHA. (The HHA is the most cost-effective method of health assessment. The price ranges from $5 to $50, but the average charge for the better ones is $15.)

The main advantage of the HHA is that it can identify health hazards years before a disease might show up on a routine physical examination or begin to cause symptoms. It has been estimated that HHAs can achieve a level of accuracy in predicting health hazards of 85% to 90%. The same percentage holds for the probability of preventing a specific disease if the individual eliminates all the risk factors by appropriate behavioral change. The HHA does not, however, suggest that an individual can alter a risk factor over which he or she has no control.

Throughout our lives we move back and forth on a wellness-illness continuum. There are levels or degrees of wellness just as there are with illness. The continuum runs from high-level wellness (H) on one end to terminal illness and death (D) on the other. This concept can be diagrammed:

H   D

Our behavioral patterns determine where on the continuum we spend most of our lives. This does not mean that all illness is self-induced or that all accidents are self-inflicted. Rather, it means, as I have repeatedly stated, that 50% of our illnesses and accidents can be prevented by appropriate change in individual lifestyles.

As I have also noted before, physicians traditionally have confined their activities to the illness side of the continuum. The physician becomes interested in the individual at the onset (O) of an illness.

H	O	Illness	D

Physicians' ministrations are designed to return individuals, free of disease, to the point on the continuum where they were picked up. Very few physicians have the time, interest, or skills required to help people attain a higher level of wellness once the specific disease is cured. That is, physicians do not operate between H and O on the continuum—the area of wellness.

H	Wellness	O	Illness	D

When you become ill—let us say you have lung cancer, as an extreme example—you come in contact with the medical care system at a point somewhere between O and D. If you are lucky, you come early enough near point O so that the cancer is still localized and you may be cured. Your physician is able to return you to point O. But that happens in only 10% of the cases. Unfortunately, in the other 90%, the physician can only hope to delay the inevitable progression to point D.

Health promotion programs are designed to reach you at a point on the continuum between H and O, while you are still well, before the onset of any disease. An HHA at this time can make you aware of the risk of developing a specific disease. You need never get to point O for that disease *if* you eliminate the risk factors. And even more important, you can get to point H and stay there by adopting a healthy lifestyle—by practicing wellness.

The onset of most diseases is simultaneous with the appearance of signs (Sg) and symptoms (Sm) of that disease. That is, most diseases do not have an asymptomatic interval between their onset and the appearance of symptoms. This can be diagrammed:

H	Wellness	O	Illness	D
		Sg		
		Sm		

As I mentioned in Chapter 19, there are only a few diseases for which early detection can make a difference as far as outcome is concerned, medically or economically. Glaucoma, diabetes, high blood pressure, syphilis, tuberculosis, and some cancers (especially breast, cervix, colon, and prostate) can exist for some time before they cause symptoms. It is this asymptomatic phase of these few diseases that has led to the medical rituals of annual, preemployment, and insurance physicals.

For years, the American Cancer Society's slogan was an annual check and a checkup. Unfortunately, lung cancer, which kills more people than any other kind, is usually incurable by the time the first signs of the disease show up as a spot on the chest X-ray film.* Although it does have an asymptomatic phase, it is not routinely detected on physical examination.

The onset of most diseases with an asymptomatic phase can be diagrammed:

H	Wellness	*O*	Illness	*D*
		Sg	*Sm*	

This indicates that signs (Sg) are present at the onset of the disease, but symptoms (Sm) develop sometime later. The interval between Sg and Sm represents the asymptomatic phase of the disease.

The annual physical is simply a search for signs of asymptomatic disease. Its effectiveness is restricted to the few diseases mentioned above and only for the relatively short time interval between Sg and Sm (the asymptomatic phase).

The HHA, however, with its search for behavioral risk factors, can be effective years before the onset of a disease process. Its area of effectiveness stretches between *H* and *O* on the wellness-illness continuum:

H	Wellness	*O*	Illness	*D*
	Risk Factors	*Sg*	*Sm*	

Area of effectiveness of the HHA:

H		*O*

---

* The American Cancer Society, in its annual report on the status of cancer, announced that 430,000 Americans will die of cancer in 1982—1,180 persons every day, one every 73 seconds. About 111,000 of these deaths, more than 25% of the total, will be from lung cancer. Lung cancer is increasing at a faster rate than any other cancer, especially in women; there will be 129,000 additional cases in 1982. Only 9 out of every 100 lung cancer patients live five years or more following diagnosis. Unlike other forms of cancer, there has been little improvement in medicine's ability to cure lung cancer, once it has been diagnosed. "The irony of this situation is that lung cancer is among the most preventable of all diseases," said a spokesman for the American Cancer Society. "The best way to avoid getting it is to give up cigarettes."

Contrast this with the limited area of effectiveness of the annual physical:

$$\frac{O}{Sg \qquad Sm}$$

When the effectiveness and the cost of these two approaches to health assessment are compared, the conclusion is obvious: The HHA is much more cost effective. The HHA is twenty times less costly ($15 versus $300) and its effectiveness can be measured in applicability years before the onset of disease, compared with weeks after the onset of illness.

In 1980, in *Diagnosis,* Dr. Jack Hall reported the results of comparing the HHA with the standard history and physical in terms of detecting health problems of which the individual was unaware. The HHA found 6.41 problems per patient compared with the 2.47 problems per patient detected by the routine history and physical.

It should be clear why the HHA has become the method used in most health promotion programs to assess the health status of the individual participants and to make them aware of the hazards in their lifestyles.

But let me clarify a point. All my praise of the HHA should not be interpreted to mean that history-taking and physical exams by a physician should be put on the shelf with the leeches and old apothecary jars of nux vomica. On the contrary, no diagnosis can ever be made without these tools. What I am condemning is the annual physical as the primary means of health assessment for the prevention of disease. It is ineffective and too costly. I am advocating the HHA as a mass screening instrument in preventive medicine. Even more, I believe it should be used as part of the routine practice of medicine to make the individual aware of specific health hazards, particularly with those chronic diseases that can be prevented only by adopting an appropriate lifestyle years before their usual onset.

If we are to be at all successful in preventing heart disease and lung cancer, for instance, we must get the message to the teenager who is contemplating smoking. "DON'T START," we would like to yell. Or, if you have started, "STOP NOW, before it's too late." But teenagers are concerned with now, not what may happen at age forty-five; that's too far into the future to worry about. What does it mean to say that the next few years may be all the smoke it takes to light the long fuse of heart disease and the equally long one of lung cancer? (We know that just a few months' exposure to asbestos can kill you twenty years from now.) "PLEASE STOP!" we keep on crying.

But yelling won't get them to stop. We have to show them specifically how smoking affects their bodies, in terms they can understand. Early use of the HHA as part of the educational process in our schools could turn the tide. Recent experiments are encouraging, but they have also shown that education alone will not succeed. Schoolchildren need a supportive environment as well as knowledge of healthy behavior, especially if they are to resist peer pressure to adopt an unhealthy lifestyle.

The American Health Foundation's "Know Your Body" program has been tested, revised, and retested since 1974 in New York City schools. The program started with an HHA, followed by a general health education course as part of the regular curriculum. By itself, this program was ineffective. So a new tactic was tried. High-risk students, identified by the HHA, were given special small-group sessions. They learned about coping with social situations that frequently cause anxiety in teenagers and about the techniques advertisers employ to get people to use their products. Then they role-played making their own decisions about smoking, drinking, and how to drive a car. In the test school, this program reduced the incidence of new smoking by 75% during the study year.

The Smoking Digest, a booklet put out by the Public Health Service and National Institutes of Health, reports a rapid increase in female teenage smokers. Between 1968 and 1974, girls moved from smoking only half as frequently as boys to full equality. This rise is paralleled by a marked increase in lung cancer in women. Although 92% of teenagers believe that smoking is harmful to health, 85% believe they will quit in five years. Yet, 60% of teenage smokers have tried to quit and failed, and 72% of women smokers aged eighteen to thirty-five have been unsuccessful at quitting.

Teenage smoking can act as a trigger mechanism, setting off a chain of events that leads to arteriosclerosis, the precursor of heart disease (the leading cause of death) and stroke (the third leading cause). Carbon monoxide, the most poisonous of the gaseous components of cigarettes, damages the walls of arteries, making them more permeable. Fluid then accumulates beneath the lining cells (this is called edema), and this area becomes the site of the deposits of cholesterol seen in arteriosclerosis.

What we have is a typical example of how unhealthy habits lead to bodily changes that are the precursors of disease. Since these bodily changes occur before the onset of a clinical disease, in most instances they can be reversed and the disease prevented. Thus, *these bodily changes are also considered risk factors*. Although they cannot be identified as early as a behavioral risk factor, they are probably more significant because they confirm that behavior has already damaged the body and the onset of disease is more certain.

Let us take a heavy smoker who has a diet high in saturated animal fats, is under a great deal of stress at work, and gets little exercise. Eventually, this lifestyle will cause specific bodily changes: an increase in blood pressure, an elevated serum cholesterol, and a decreased vital capacity (the ability of the lungs to exchange carbon dioxide for oxygen). An HHA will identify the unhealthy behaviors, but other tests are needed to uncover the bodily changes: physiometric measurement to detect the elevated blood pressure, blood chemistry to show the high serum cholesterol, and spirometry (a breathing test) to pick up the impaired pulmonary function.

The identification of these bodily changes is usually done through multiphasic screening by nonphysician personnel. The findings are put into the computer, along with the results of the HHA questionnaire. The output then gives a more sophisticated assessment of an individual's risk factors.

Multiphasic health testing also identifies those risk factors that are not behavioral in origin, once they have caused bodily changes to occur. These are the risk factors that are primarily biological (hereditary) or environmental in origin. Still, as I mentioned in the previous chapter, they may be augmented or modified by behavior.

These two tools, the HHA and multiphasic health testing, should be incorporated as part of periodic health assessments all of us should receive throughout our entire lifetime, beginning in childhood.

In 1977, writing in the *New England Journal of Medicine*, Dr. Lester Breslow and Anne R. Somers introduced a new, practical approach to preventive medicine called the "Lifetime Health-Monitoring Program" (LHMP). At the time, Breslow was dean of the UCLA School of Public Health and Somers, a well-respected health economist, was a professor in the Department of Environmental and Community Medicine, College of Medicine and Dentistry of New Jersey, Rutgers Medical School.

Breslow and Somers challenged the medical profession to give up the annual checkup and approach prevention by focusing on specific chronic illness and emphasizing major risk factors—cigarette smoking, obesity, elevated blood lipid levels, hypertension, and alcoholism. They proposed a program that would be relevant and cost effective for specific populations at specific age levels. They felt that this program should be incorporated into medical practice to reconcile public health and private practice goals.

The LHMP is a series of packages of effective individual preventive procedures for various age groups that have different health needs, problems, and changing lifestyles. Breslow and Somers divided the lifespan into ten periods, based on different needs: fetal and perinatal, infancy (first year of life), preschool age (one to five), school age (six to eleven), adolescence (twelve to seventeen), young adult (eighteen to twenty-four), young middle age (twenty-five to thirty-nine), older middle age (forty to fifty-nine), elderly (sixty to seventy-four), and old age (seventy-five and over).

For each of the ten age groups, a set of distinct health goals and professional services was described. Here are some representative examples.*

Preschool Child (One to Five)
  Health goals:
  1. To facilitate the child's optimal physical, emotional, and social growth and development.
  2. To begin the process of socialization through happy and effective family relations and gradual introduction to school and other facets of the outside world.
  Professional services:
  1. Two professional visits with the healthy child and mother (ideally, the father also) at two to three years of age and at school entry for compliance with immunization schedule, and for observation and counseling about nutrition, activity, vision, hearing, speech, dental health, accident prevention, and general physical, emotional, and social development.
  2. For special high-risk groups, blood tests for anemia, lead poisoning, and tuberculosis skin tests.
Young Adult (eighteen to twenty-four)
  Health goals:
  1. To facilitate transition from dependent adolescence to mature independent adulthood with maximal physical, mental, and emotional resources.
  2. To achieve useful employment and maximum capacity for a healthy marriage, parenthood, and social relations.
  Professional services:
  1. One professional visit with the healthy adult, including complete physical examination, tetanus booster if not received within the previous ten years, tests for syphilis, gonorrhea, malnutrition, cholesterol, and hypertension, and medical and behavioral history. This visit should be provided upon entrance into college, the armed forces, the first full-time job, and definitely before marriage.

* Lester Breslow and Anne R. Somers, "Lifetime Health Monitoring Program."

2. Health education and individual counseling, as needed, for nutrition, exercise, study, career, job, occupational hazards and problems, sex, contraception, marriage and family relations, alcohol, drugs, smoking, and driving.
3. Dental examination and prophylaxis every two years.

Older Middle Age (forty to fifty-nine)

Health goals:

1. To prolong the period of maximum physical energy and optimum mental and social activity, including menopausal adjustment.
2. To detect as early as possible any of the major chronic diseases, including hypertension, heart disease, diabetes, and cancer, as well as vision, hearing, and dental impairments.

Professional services:

1. Four professional visits with the healthy person, once every five years, with complete physical examination and medical history, tests for specific chronic conditions, appropriate immunizations, and counseling regarding changing nutritional needs, physical activities, occupation, sex, marital and parental problems, and use of cigarettes, alcohol, and other drugs.
2. For those over fifty, annual screening tests for hypertension, obesity, and certain cancers. Otherwise, specific screening every two to five years.
3. Annual dental prophylaxis.

Specific screening procedures: (These are ones I would suggest; others may differ. They may be carried out by nonphysician personnel.)

Suspected disease or condition	Screening procedure
Intervals of two to three years	
Malnutrition, including obesity	Height/weight, nutrition and activity history*
Hypertension and assoc. conditions	Blood pressure, urinalysis*
Cervical cancer	Papanicolaou smear
Colon cancer	Stool for blood*
Breast cancer	Breast self-examination
Lung cancer	Smoking history
Endometrial cancer of uterus	History of postmenopausal bleeding*

* Once a year over fifty.

Intervals of five years

Coronary artery disease	Cholesterol, triglycerides, HDLP, LDLP (high- and low-density lipoproteins), electrocardiogram
Alcoholism; cirrhosis	Drinking history; if positive, liver function studies (blood chemistry)
Anemia	Hemoglobin
Diabetes	Fasting and one-hour p.c. (postprandial) blood sugar
Glaucoma	Tonometry (tension of eyeball)
Chronic obstructive pulmonary disease (COPD); emphysema	Spirometry (breathing test) if impaired function, chest X ray
Lung cancer	Chest X ray (heavy smokers only)*
Tuberculosis	PPD (skin test); if positive, chest X ray
Syphilis	VDRL (blood test)
Vision defect	Audiogram
Hearing defect	Refraction

Note: These screening procedures can be performed most cost effectively by an HHA ($15) and an automated multiphasic health testing ($25 to $50). Most insurance agents can guide you to reliable multiphasic health testing centers in your community. Your local hospital may provide such a service, ask your doctor. Results of these tests should be sent to your physician and you should set up an appointment for a counseling session (not a physical exam, unless there are positive findings on the screening results).

Old Age (seventy-five and up)
 Health goals:
1. To prolong period of effective activity and ability to live independently; to avoid institutionalization so far as possible.
2. To minimize inactivity and discomfort from chronic conditions.
3. When illness is terminal, to assure as little physical and mental distress as possible and to provide emotional support to patient and family.
 Professional services:

* Once a year over fifty.

1. Professional visit at least once a year, including complete physical examination, medical and behavioral history, and professional counseling regarding changing nutritional requirements, limitations on activity and mobility, and living arrangements.
2. Annual immunization against influenza (unless allergic to the vaccine).
3. Periodic dental and podiatric treatment as needed.
4. For low-income and other persons not sick enough to be institutionalized but not well enough to cope entirely alone, counseling regarding sheltered housing, health visitors, home health services, day care and recreational centers, meals-on-wheels, and other measures designed to help them remain in their own homes and be as independent as possible.
5. Professional assistance with family relations and preparations for death, if needed.

Similar health goals and professional services are suggested for the other age groups. Taking professional visits, for example, we find: for infants (first year), one recommended visit immediately following birth and four later visits; for preschoolers, two visits; for schoolchildren, two visits; for adolescents, one visit; for young adults, one visit; for middle-aged adults, six visits; for the elderly, one visit every two years; for the very old, at least one visit per year. All this adds up to about twenty-five periodic health evaluations over an average lifetime of seventy-six years. If average cost was $100 per professional visit, the total would be only $2,500 for a lifetime, or about $33 a year. This same $2,500 would cover only seven annual physicals of the executive type at today's prices.

At $33 per year, we could provide every man, woman, and child in the United States with a Lifetime Health-Monitoring Program at an annual cost of $8.25 billion. This figure is only 3% of our present total annual health expenditure of $287 billion. Such an emphasis on prevention could cut the incidence of disease by half and shave at least $100 billion off our annual health expenditures.

In an editorial in the December 1981 issue of the *Journal of Public Health Policy*, Milton Terris substantiates these estimates:

Expanded public health control programs could bring the death rate from cerebrovascular disease down to a third or a quarter of the 1978 rate of 79 per 100,000 population. The ischemic heart disease rate could be lowered to about 40% of the 1978 rate of 294, to approximate the current rates in Switzerland and Italy. We need to emulate the United Kingdom and lower our cirrhosis mortality rate of 14 to approach their rate of only 4 per 100,000. Deaths from other major diseases, such as lung cancer and chronic obstructive lung disease, should decrease by at least 50% as intensified public health programs accelerate the decline in cigarette smoking. And a really serious effort to control accidents, poisoning, and violence would lower the toll from these major causes of death by at least a third. These goals are realistic and feasible; they can not only be achieved but surpassed.*

Adoption of the Lifetime Health-Monitoring Program by the medical profession could hasten such an improvement. An ounce of prevention today is worth a $100 billion of cure.

It will take more than wishful thinking, however, to move the Medical Establishment. It will take all of us, as knowledgeable consumers of health care, to bring this about. The first step is for each of us to identify our own health hazards and reclaim responsibility for our own health.

What you can do right now is to obtain a Health Hazard Appraisal. Several HHAs are on the market. I prefer either the four-page or eight-page questionnaire from Medical Datamation, Bellevue, Ohio 44811 (telephone: 800-537-2893). The original Health Hazard Appraisal can be obtained from Methodist Hospital, Indianapolis, Indiana 46202 (317-924-6411); this is a two-page questionnaire. Complete information on HHAs and a list of additional sources can be obtained from the Centers for Disease Control, Bureau of Health Education, 1600 Clifton Road, N.E., Atlanta, Georgia 30333 (404-329-3415).

Samples of the four-page and the eight-page questionnaires from Medical Datamation appear in the Appendix. There are also examples of computer printouts and feedback to the individual. Medical Datamation calls its HHA a Health Risk Index; it has been augmented with a Lifestyle Index, which includes an analysis of the individual's nutrition, exercise, and stress level. The eight-page questionnaire also includes a health history report. This report is designed for your doctor, and it is an excellent way of making sure the doctor has all the information you want him or her to have about you.

At this writing, the cost of the Medical Datamation four-page HHA is $12; the eight-page version is $15. These costs include the questionnaire, computer processing, mailing, personal feedback reports for you and your physician, and educational booklets relating to all health hazards identified.

After you have obtained the results of your HHA, call your doctor for an appointment. Take the reports with you and discuss them. This is also a good time to discuss your own plan for lifetime health monitoring. You will soon find out how interested your doctor is in your health.

* Milton Terris, Editorial.

CHAPTER 24

Preventing Disease by Risk Factor Intervention

IMAGINE you now have the results of your Health Hazard Appraisal in hand and you are off to discuss your health risks with your doctor, whom we'll call Dr. Samuel Abel. You wonder what Dr. Abel's opinion will be and how you will respond to his reaction. Remember, as you enter your doctor's office: You've come to discuss *your* health—what is good for you, no one else. You are here as a client, not as a patient.

What will happen? There are three general responses you might anticipate. The most deflating is condescension, so let's deal with that first. Dr. Abel puts on his glasses, leans back in his swivel chair, and gives your HHA report a cursory reading. Expect at least three "umm-humms" during this period. He then puts down the report and comments, "Very interesting. But you realize this has never been shown to be of value in clinical trials."

"Have they done any clinical trials?" you ask.

"Not that I know of. But if it were of any value, I'd have heard of it. Now you just take off your clothes and get up on the table, and I'll examine you. Come on now."

Take this response as your cue to reclaim your own life. Go back to Chapter 19 and reread the part about how to find a family doctor.

Another response, although the least likely, is total affirmation of the HHA. There's an outside chance that Dr. Abel will believe that risk factor intervention is the key to preventing disease and will be willing to act as your counselor as you plan for your own wellness. He wants to set up a Lifetime Health-Monitoring Program for you, without your asking. You are understandably speechless—but overjoyed. You are well on your way.

Between these two extremes is the Dr. Abel you will most likely encounter—the physician who knows very little about the concept but who finds the idea stimulating and interesting and is honest enough to tell you so. I would stay with this Dr. Abel; you can learn together. Tell him how he can send for his own HHA. And give him the reference to Breslow and

Somers' article on their LHMP (see the Bibliography). This should impress him.

The first help you would like to get from Dr. Abel is his opinion on whether or not your identified risk factors require further assessment at this time. Is multiphasic health testing indicated to determine if bodily changes have already taken place? Is a physical exam indicated? Should any special tests be done? Since the objective is to determine your exact health status, further testing may be necessary. The result should be a complete understanding of your health status and an identification of your health hazards for the next five to ten years.

Now that you've identified hazards, what's the next step? You need to set your health goals for the ensuing five years, with interim objectives to help you along to your long-range goals.

Let us suppose that you are a middle-aged man and the following risk factors are identified: You smoke two packs of cigarettes per day; you are twenty pounds overweight; you exercise only on weekends when you play eighteen holes of golf; your blood pressure is elevated to 165/92 (when 140/80 would be normal); your serum cholesterol is high (285, when 175 would be normal); and your level of stress is moderately high. Dr. Abel thinks you should have an electrocardiogram (EKG). It shows slight left ventricular hypertrophy (thickening of the wall of the heart) but is otherwise normal.

Most of the time you feel great, you tell the doctor. You're a little sluggish at times, but usually you have all the energy you need. You are really surprised that for your actual age of forty-five your HHA gave you an appraisal age of sixty and a life expectancy of only twelve years. This has scared the hell out of you and you are willing to do almost anything. You still feel like a young man and you certainly don't plan to die at age fifty-seven. You want Dr. Abel's help.

Dr. Abel reminds you that the HHA also indicated that you could achieve a health age of forty-three and expect to live to age seventy-eight. That's thirty-three more years—a lot better. All you have to do is change most of your habits. You might feel all right at present, but you have a high risk of developing coronary heart disease. According to the Framingham Risk Score, you have a probability of 426 out of 1,000, or a 42.6% likelihood of developing coronary heart disease within eight years unless you change a lot of behaviors.

You take his word for it, hoping that some day he will explain what the Framingham Risk Score is. But for now, you want to get on with it.

What is your goal for the next five years? That's easy: to achieve that health age at which you can expect to live to be seventy-eight. But that is going to be hard. To reach that goal, you have a whole list of objectives to accomplish. You had better write them down.

1. Stop smoking in two months.
2. Lose twenty pounds in four months.
3. Exercise every day for twenty minutes, starting tomorrow.
4. Get blood pressure down to 140/80 in six months.
5. Reduce serum cholesterol to less than 200 in three months.
6. Learn how to deal with stress, starting now.

Are these realistic goals? Yes. And you will notice Dr. Abel made you put a time frame on each objective. If you agree with this program, sign it. Make this list a contract with yourself (and your physician). It has been shown that this approach will increase your chances of success.

A couple of the objectives overlap, Dr. Abel explains. You will be able to achieve two for the effort of one. Losing twenty pounds and lowering your serum cholesterol can be accomplished with the same diet. If you learn how to deal with stress, you'll probably lower your blood pressure in the process. It's worth trying before you resort to medication.

You can rewrite your objectives, then, for brevity and clarity. (Four objectives are easier to accomplish than six.)

1. Stop smoking within two months.
2. Change eating habits so as to lose twenty pounds in four months and to reduce serum cholesterol to less than 200 in three months.
3. Exercise every day for twenty minutes, starting tomorrow (this will also help keep weight down).
4. Learn how to deal with stress, starting now, and get blood pressure down to 140/80 in six months.

The next morning you reread your contract with yourself. Working on that list of objectives seemed so easy last night in the doctor's office; now you have some doubts. He told you that changing your lifestyle would be difficult, but you didn't think it would be so hard to even start. The status quo seems so comfortable this morning.

Hold it! You need to do two things immediately. First, find a friend and then reread your HHA. You need support to make these changes. Your spouse might be the ideal person to work with you. The supporting environment of a loving family makes change easier and can help you maintain your new patterns. Share your HHA report with at least one person who loves you. And to help dispel your doubts, let me tell you about the increasing evidence that this concept really works.

In 1965, the Human Population Laboratory of Alameda County, California, decided to follow the health practices of a representative sample of the county's adult population for several years. It chose 6,928 adults for the study. Their physical health status and their longevity were monitored over nine and a half years in relation to the practice of seven common good health habits:

1. Never smokes cigarettes.
2. Has regular physical activity.
3. Maintains proper weight.
4. Uses alcohol only in moderation.
5. Gets seven to eight hours sleep every night.
6. Eats three meals daily, but never eats between meals.
7. Always eats breakfast.

The findings of the study were very significant:

- The physical health status of those following all seven good health practices was consistently the same as for those thirty years younger who followed few or none of these practices. This was independent of age, sex, and income level.
- The physical health status was consistently proportional to the number of these practices followed; seven was higher than six, six higher than five, etc.
- The mortality rate for men following all seven practices was 57% lower than that for all men in the study and 72% lower than for men who followed fewer than three of these health practices.
- The mortality rate for women who followed all seven health practices was 38% lower than that for all women in the study and 57% lower than that for women who practiced fewer than three.*

The conclusion is obvious: Following good health habits favors longevity and high physical health status.

And what about that Framingham Risk Score? The risk factors for coronary heart disease (also referred to as atherosclerotic or ischemic heart disease) were largely determined by a lengthy epidemiological study of the disease in Framingham, Massachusetts, in the 1960s. Dr. Donald S. Frederickson, director of the National Institutes of Health, writing in *Harrison's Principles of Internal Medicine*, lists the risk factors for this disease in the order of their importance for American males:

1. Hyperlipidemia (elevated cholesterol, triglycerides, and/or low-density lipoproteins)

---

* Findings summarized from: L. Breslow and J. Enstrom, "Persistence of Health Habits and Their Relationship to Mortality."

2. Hypertension (high blood pressure)
3. Cigarette smoking
4. Diabetes mellitus
5. Physical inactivity
6. Obesity
7. Emotional stress
8. Positive family history of premature atherosclerosis

The Framingham study clearly shows that combinations of the first four of these risk factors, plus an EKG finding of left ventricular hypertrophy, have a compounding or cumulative effect that increases the probability of developing cardiovascular disease thirtyfold within eight years as each risk factor is added.

Thus, a forty-five-year-old male with normal blood pressure, who does not smoke, has a normal cholesterol of 185, and has no glucose intolerance, will have a probability of only 22/1000 of developing coronary heart disease. But if his blood pressure goes up to 195 systolic and all other risk factors stay normal, his risk increases to 84/1000. If he smokes, the risk increases to 138/1000. If he develops glucose intolerance (a bodily change that is a precursor to diabetes), his risk climbs to 226/1000. If his cholesterol reaches 335, the risk increases to 550/1000, and when his EKG shows left ventricular hypertrophy, the risk becomes thirty times as great as it was originally—778/1000, or a 77.8% likelihood of developing the disease.

This cumulative effect of compounding several risk factors also occurs in women but to a lesser degree because of their premenopausal hormonal protection from atherosclerosis and coronary heart disease. Even at age fifty-five, there appears to be some residual protection. For example, a fifty-five-year-old male whose only coronary risk factor is a high systolic blood pressure of 180 has 90/1000 chances of having a coronary. If his cholesterol reaches 335, the chances increase to 188/1000. But his female counterpart, aged fifty-five, with the same systolic pressure of 180 will have only 38/1000 chances, and if her cholesterol reaches 335 this only increases her risk to 94/1000, half that of the man.

But can risk factor intervention reverse the process and reduce the chance of developing a disease?

The answer is yes. Risk factor intervention does reduce the risk of developing a disease. The best evidence we have to date relates to smoking as a risk factor for lung cancer. An epidemiological study of over a million ex-smokers, who had smoked less than a pack per day, showed that when they stopped smoking there was a gradual but immediate decrease in their risk of lung cancer, to the point where in ten years it was the same as if they had never smoked.* For those who smoked over a pack per day, the risk did not begin to decrease until five years after they stopped, and after ten years it was still slightly higher than for those who did not smoke. Heavy smokers (more than two packs per day) had an increased mortality for the first year after they stopped because they usually stopped for a serious illness.

In Chapter 19, I mentioned the 22% decrease in deaths from coronary heart disease between 1968 and 1978, which followed the health kick that spontaneously erupted in America during the 1960s. Let me repeat: We jogged; we switched from foods high in saturated animal fats to unsaturated vegetable oils low in cholesterol. Several million stopped smoking after the Surgeon General's first report in 1964 (and the percentage of males smoking dropped from 52% in 1964 to 39% in 1975). In addition, a higher percentage of those with hypertension came under treatment. This change was strictly an American phenomenon, one not seen in other parts of the world. And the decreased mortality rate was seen only in the United States.

What happened was that we inadvertently eliminated five of the six leading risk factors for coronary heart disease. And the mortality rate dropped 22%.

Public health physicians, and especially epidemiologists, became excited about the possibility of using risk factor intervention as a preventive strategy. Two longitudinal studies of controlled clinical trials of risk factor intervention were started in the early 1970s. The researchers hoped to determine the most effective site of intervention—within traditional medical practice or on a community-wide basis. They also wanted to find the best ways to motivate individuals to change behavior. Another goal was to determine the extent to which risk factors could be reversed. It was most important, however, to discover if reduction in risk factors resulted in decreased incidence of a disease.

The first of these clinical trials, still in progress, is the Multiple Risk Factor Intervention Trial (MRFIT). Sponsored by the National Heart, Lung, and Blood Institute of NIH, this study has involved twenty medical centers in a cooperative randomized clinical trial on 12,866 male volunteers aged thirty-five to fifty-seven. The men were selected as high-risk individuals according to the Framingham Risk Score, which identifies high serum cholesterol, high blood pressure, and cigarette smoking as three

* E.C. Hammond, "Smoking in Relation to Death Rates of One Million, Men and Women."

main risk factors for coronary heart disease. Simultaneous intervention aimed at these three risk factors is being conducted on an individual and group basis. Results of the study are expected in 1983.

Another clinical trial has been undertaken by the Department of Cardiology, Stanford University Medical School. It is known as the Stanford Heart Disease Prevention Program. Three cities in northern California were selected for a community-based intervention trial using the same three risk factors as the MRFIT program. One city was used as a control, with no intervention. Mass media educational programs were beamed at the other two cities. In one, the high-risk groups were also isolated and intensive interventions were directed at those individuals.

Early results show a 15% to 20% reduction in these risk factors in the two trial cities' total population and a 30% reduction in the isolated high-risk group. An ongoing study involving five cities is now under way.

A similar program is being tried in North Karelia, Finland, the community with the highest incidence of coronary heart disease and stroke in that country. The program is also intervening in cigarette smoking, high cholesterol levels, and hypertension. Preliminary reports showed a reduction of all three risk factors and a reduction of the incidence of stroke in males from 3.6/1000 in 1972 to 1.9/1000 in 1975; in females from 2.8 to 1.8/1000.

So, you see, it really does work. Now, how do we get you started? We don't—you have to do it yourself. But there are many individuals and groups waiting to help you whenever you ask.

In fact, recent research into the applications of social learning theory is coming up with new ways to help people change. Central to social learning theory is the concept that our psychological functioning is determined by the continuous interplay among three separate factors: our behavior, our cognitive knowledge and belief system, and our immediate environment—as A. Bandura explains in a 1978 issue of *American Psychologist*.

In other words, our behavior is influenced by people around us and by what we know and believe. We anticipate the consequences of our actions from those around us (they will be offended if I smoke) and from our knowledge (that article I read showed smoking causes lung cancer). At the same time our behavior is continuously affecting our immediate environment (I don't smoke, and I choose friends who don't smoke; there aren't even any ashtrays in my house) and our cognitive system (now that I've stopped smoking and can feel the benefits, I really believe it's lethal for everybody).

Bandura has also shown that understanding the ways we ordinarily go about managing our behavior is essential for changing and maintaining new habits. Simply stated, we begin with self-observation of our actions; then we judge them by our personal standards, by the degree to which we value the activity as worthwhile, and by the standards of society we have accepted as valid for our lives. If the behavior is deemed to affect our welfare and self-esteem, our response is one of reward or punishment (self-imposed). Otherwise, we ignore the behavior as irrelevant.

Our previous behavior is continuously used as the reference point for judging our ongoing performance. Previous attainments influence our performance appraisal by altering our standards. After a given level of performance is achieved, for instance, it is no longer challenging, and new self-satisfactions are sought in a train of progressive improvement.

The best way to modify or change our behavior is to first understand how the change can benefit us. We need to increase our knowledge of the consequences of the change we are contemplating. Then we need to spell out a series of short-term objectives and long-term goals. These goals must be considered important for our welfare and self-esteem. We must choose our own approach to the new behavior, compatible with our belief system. And there have to be meaningful rewards as recognition of our accomplishment.*

We are the only ones who can control and change our behavior. But, by using these principles, we are capable of changing any behavior we want to change. Just follow the simple steps:

1. Identify your health hazard. The Health Hazard Appraisal is the most cost-effective way to accomplish this step. It will also identify the specific risk factors in terms of behaviors you should change.
2. Increase your knowledge of the problem. Through reading or in consultation with your doctor, begin to understand the consequences of not making a change and the benefits you will receive from the change.
3. Make the commitment to make the change. Write a contract with yourself. Spell out exactly what you want to accomplish and why. Be sure to specify a realistic time frame. Sign it.
4. Chart your behavior in relation to the problem. Keep a diary for one, two, or three days, even a week if it takes that long to establish the pattern of your behavior. If you are trying to correct overeating, discover what you eat, when you eat it, and how you felt before and after

---

* A good example of the application of this theory is a smoking cessation program found in the Appendix to this book. This program is based on one advocated by the U.S. Department of Health and Human Services, but it has been augmented and the format has been changed according to my own experience as I stopped smoking.

you ate it. Begin to think how you could break the pattern and substitute healthier activities instead of having that snack.

5. Plan your approach to the change. Establish your long-range goal (or goals). Write it down. Then spell out a series of short-term objectives you can deal with gradually to eventually reach your goal. Write them down, with a realistic time frame. Remember, your goals must be considered important to your welfare and self-esteem. Your approach must be compatible with your belief system. Set a starting date. Share your plan with your family or a close friend who is willing to give you moral support; try to find someone who has had the problem and has overcome it. Start on your first objective.

6. Reward yourself. Don't wait until you have attained your goal (although you should also plan a big reward for that time). Every day congratulate yourself on the progress you have made. Share your pleasure with the person giving you moral support. If you encounter a snag in your plan, change the plan. Just don't become discouraged; you may have been unrealistic in setting objectives. Rethink your whole plan; renew your commitment. See how far you have already come.

7. Keep on rewarding yourself. When you have reached your goal have that big celebration you planned. Notice what a better person you are and feel good about it. Plan periodic celebrations of your victory.

CHAPTER 25

Beyond Prevention:
Toward Optimal Wellness

THE GREATEST MOVE toward health promotion has been made outside the Medical Establishment by men and women who grew up with the fitness groundswell of the 1960s. These individuals have embraced wellness as a way of life and with their healthy lifestyle have inadvertently eliminated the risk factors for the leading causes of death in the United States. They have arrived at the same point as those who are interested in the prevention of disease, but from the opposite direction.

From the start, their approach has been one of health promotion, not disease prevention. Their goal is to achieve the highest level of wellness. They believe that if wellness is practiced as a way of life early enough, we will stay well. They embrace the definition of health as the optimal achievable state of well-being in body, mind, and spirit.

Although these individuals are part of a movement that is gaining momentum in America, they are not formally organized. They are not a religion. They are interested in the whole individual, but not in the same context as the holistic movement (which is a new approach to treatment of disease and not a promotion of health).

The people I am talking about are a group of unique individuals who look at health in the same way. And health is one of the most important aspects of their lives. They believe that if they are healthy, then wealthy and wise will take care of themselves.

They read a great deal and have spawned a new literature on the subject of health promotion. They attend wellness-oriented meetings to learn more about wellness from each other, not to form organizations. They are very supportive of one another, however, and many know each other on a first-name basis. It is rare to hear them address individuals by titles, such as Mister or Miss or Doctor, or by last names.

Those I have met are very loving people. They embrace one another openly and without embarrassment. They are always willing to share knowledge and experience. They have no designated leaders, and no one seems to be trying to become one. They have no dogma; everyone seeks his or her own elements of wellness. The approaches are diverse—whatever works for the individual is what counts.

They are a mixed group—men and women, old and young, black and white, of Asian and European origin, Catholic and Protestant, Jew and Gentile, Republican and Democrat, gay and straight, rich and poor, blue collar and white collar, from the city, suburbs, and rural areas. But they are different from most of us in five basic ways.

First, they have taken responsibility for their own lives and especially for their health. They use the Medical Establishment wisely—as clients, not as compliant patients, when they are well. If they do become sick, they trust and cooperate with the physician to reach their mutual goal.

Second, they have an awareness of nutrition. They realize that we are, literally, what we eat. The body is constantly replacing its cells; what we eat this month becomes our muscle, bones, and blood vessels next month. They read the labels on all packaged foods and, therefore, rarely buy them. Instead, they prefer to eat foods as close to their natural state as possible, which they prepare themselves. They never eat junk food with its high sugar, salt, and fat content.

Third, they have acquired the skills to manage stress. They use stress for productivity and creativity in their lives. They also know how to deal with nonproductive stress; for them, it almost never becomes distress.

Fourth, they are sensitive to their environment. As responsible citizens, they support pollution control and oppose the contamination of our food chain with chemical contaminants. They walk lightly on the earth. But their main concern is their personal environment, the one they create for themselves—their personal space, family, friends; their hearth.

Finally, they are physically fit. They consider the body the dwelling place of the mind and spirit. If it is not used, it falls into disrepair (we don't recarpet a room we never use). Physical fitness brings all the other parts together; it acts as a catalyst to create the whole person.

Where do you find these people? Everywhere you go. There is usually a higher concentration in health food stores, spas, parks, gardens, and wilderness areas. But they are all over. There are probably a few in your church, club, or workplace.

They are easy to recognize if you look closely. Their skin glows; they don't wear heavy makeup—they don't need to. Their hair may be any color, even gray, but it has a gloss. It's not shiny, but it's never dull—and if you get to feel it, it's soft. These people's bodies are beautiful, like those of athletes. Any clothes (or none at all) look good on them. They have a bounce to their walk; they are great dancers.

I could go on and on, but I think I have drawn the picture. They are the ones you've seen and said to yourself, "I wish I could look like that." *And you can!*

No matter where you are at present on the wellness-illness continuum, you can achieve a higher level of wellness. Just keep working to the left—in an apolitical sense:

H	Wellness	O	Illness	D
		O		

If you are ill now, you will need your physician's help to get you to point O, to get free of disease. But don't stop there. You must go beyond this neutral point, where you are neither well nor ill. You must learn how to become really well and how to stay there.

If you think you are well, but live in a manner you know is unhealthy. If you smoke, drink too much, get too little exercise, are uptight most of the time, overweight. If you tire easily, if your body won't do the things your mind wants it to do. If you are irritable, hard to get along with, have lost your ambition, and your sex life is falling apart. If you are unhappy. In any of these cases, you are not really well, even if you are not sick.

If your physician is practicing risk factor intervention or if you have gotten a Health Hazard Appraisal on your own, you will probably see that you are moving to the right on the continuum, heading toward illness. It is almost impossible to stand still on the continuum. And unless you are actively following good health practices, chances are you are moving toward illness.

Risk factor intervention, no matter how you get into it (or how it finds you), will keep you from becoming ill; it will prevent disease. And it will move you to the left on the continuum. But it will not get you all the way to the highest possible level of wellness for you, point *H*. With the limited wellness resources available today, you may have to "go to *H*," health, on your own.

It would take another whole book to provide a self-help guide to high-level wellness. Fortunately for all of us, this book has already been written by Donald B. Ardell. It's called *High Level Wellness*. I will provide you with only a summary of the five dimensions of wellness it details and tell you some of the things I personally learned from and about the author.

If there were to be a Mr. Wellness U.S.A., Don Ardell would be that man. He is the personification of wellness, having the attributes I previously described. Don's background is in health planning—regulation and control of hospital beds, new technology, facilities, and equipment. After ten years, he became disenchanted because none of these activities seemed able to contain the cost of care or to have an impact on people's health.

In 1975, a friend gave him a copy of a book, also called *High Level Wellness*, written in 1961 by a physician, Herbert H. Dunn. Dunn died that same year (1975), at age 80, and Don never had the opportunity to meet him. But that little book changed his life.

The book talked about health as much more than the absence of illness. In Dunn's words, "He talked about a state wherein you actually glow with well-being, a state wherein you are 'alive clear to the tips of your fingers. You have energy to burn. You tingle with vitality. At times like these, the world is a glorious place.'" Both Dunn and Ardell call this state of well-being "high level wellness."

Don began reading all the books about health he could find. He visited all the holistic health centers, obtained leads to other individuals throughout the country who were interested in similar ideas, and began to explore and experience these new concepts and techniques on a personal level. By 1977, he had culled the chaff from his new knowledge and found the essence of wellness—the five elements he refers to as the dimensions of wellness. He then wrote his own book, using the same title Dunn had used.

I first met Don in 1977, shortly after his book was published. I, too, had become disenchanted with the Medical Establishment as it was moving further and further away from the medical needs of people and ignoring the new breakthrough in risk factor intervention, with its potential for preventing disease. I had decided to form a company to provide disease prevention programs to industry, using risk factor intervention. I anticipated that the business community would be interested in prevention as a cost-containment strategy. Thus I came to enlist Don's help in developing the details of the program.

Don introduced me to Dr. John Travis, founder of the Wellness Resource Center in Mill Valley, California. John was probably Don's chief mentor in the ways of wellness. Travis, as a physician—with an M.D. from Tufts, followed by a residency in preventive medicine and a master's degree in public health from Johns Hopkins—confirmed my belief in the necessity for this new direction in medicine.

We were in the middle of a new epidemiological revolution—and the Medical Establishment was carrying on business as usual. It was like continuing to play bridge through the bombing of Pearl Harbor. At least, that's how its apparent lack of interest made it seem.

Through personal talks and observation of Don Ardell and John Travis —as well as a course for health professionals I took at the Wellness Resource Center—I came to realize that disease prevention was not an end in itself. It was only a way station on the road to wellness.

Before we could get Hale, Inc. (the company we had formed) off the drawing board, I developed cancer of the lung. I've already indicated how this confirmed for me the importance of unhealthy behavior as the cause of disease. There is absolutely no doubt in my mind that my forty years of smoking was the direct cause of my lung cancer, even if during the last twenty years I smoked only the lowest tar and nicotine content cigarettes on the market. Although I have never agreed with those who blame victims for their disease, I must blame myself for my lung cancer; as a physician, I should have known better. (The evidence is growing, moreover, that the Medical Establishment will be contributing to at least 80% of lung cancer and 90% of coronary heart disease and stroke by continuing to ignore the importance of risk factor intervention in the prevention of these leading causes of death in America.)

So, in the spring of 1979, I found myself on the illness side of the continuum. I have already recounted my good fortune in being returned to point O. Then, I began the slow process of reclaiming my own life, becoming more well, by using the principles I had learned from John Travis and especially Don Ardell's dimensions of wellness.

There are five dimensions of wellness: self-responsibility, nutritional awareness, stress management, physical fitness, and environmental sensitivity.

Self-Responsibility

Self-responsibility is what this book is all about. My main point is that we as a nation have given up responsibility for our own health and have placed that responsibility in the hands of an authority figure, the physician. I have also tried to show that physicians have not taken on that responsibility, nor do they seem interested in doing so. Moreover, they are not interested in our health or even in our being well; they are interested in us only when we are sick. The only way we can reclaim our own health is to take back the responsibility for it.

Behavioral factors are the most important causes of our becoming ill; logically, they must be equally important in keeping us well. And behavior is the responsibility of the individual.

Our bodies are truly amazing organisms. We have built-in warning signals when something begins to go wrong. Only we can hear them—if we are attuned to our bodies. No one else can be aware of them; it is up to us.

And we are not just physical bodies, we are mind and spirit as well. Our sense of purpose and worth, our ability to love and be loved, our happiness, our total well-being, all depend on our being in control of our lives. Being in control means we have to be able to change, and self-responsibility is an essential first step in any change process.

Nutritional Awareness

Nutritional awareness is the area in which it is most difficult to achieve consensus. Everyone seems to have different advice for us; even recognized authorities do not always agree. There are certain basic areas of agreement, however, and we can use these as general guidelines. Everyone seems to agree that natural foods are better than processed foods and that when we prepare them we should try to keep them as close to their natural state as possible to preserve the nutrients. Listed below are ten guidelines for good nutrition that make sense to me. (Like everyone else, I have included my own prejudices, although I'll admit I'm not an authority on the subject.)

1. *Balance caloric intake to energy expenditure.* Most of us establish our eating habits when we are young and active. As our lives become more sedentary, we nevertheless continue with the same eating patterns. The result is obesity. You should try to remain within 10% of your nomal weight. When you begin to gain weight, you must exercise more and eat less. Chronic overeating should be considered the same as any addiction or substance abuse and should be treated the same way, including relearning of normal eating habits.

2. *Do not eat between meals.* You should establish regular patterns for meals. You may have three regular meals or six small ones, but the pattern should be based on eating when you are hungry. The amount should be determined by when you feel full, and this should in turn determine the size and frequency of your meals. (However, if you carry this rule to the extreme, you are going to drive whoever cooks in your household right up the wall, or wind up with your plate on top of your head. Remember social custom and harmony; food is not the only nourishment you need.)

3. *Always eat breakfast.* But also be careful what you eat. About the worst possible breakfast is orange juice, toast or Danish, and coffee

with cream and sugar. This high-carbohydrate meal will stimulate the pancreas to pour out insulin so that by 11:00 A.M. you are in a state of hypoglycemia (low blood sugar, similar to insulin shock). The symptoms are nervousness, depression, and, at times, extreme anxiety. It has been shown that many housewives who become alcoholics start out innocently trying to overcome the symptoms of hypoglycemia with alcohol. Alcohol does work at first, but it stimulates the pancreas to put out more insulin and in a short time the anxiety has returned, leading to a vicious circle. Hypoglycemia is especially likely if the first food to hit your stomach, breaking the nightlong fast, is orange juice. Eat whole fruit for breakfast and save the orange juice for lunch. The orange-flavored sugar-waters fortified with vitamin C are even worse.

Breakfast should be a high-protein meal. For example, a whole grain cereal, like oatmeal, with wheat germ and two tablespoons of bran for adequate fiber, is a good way to start. Try eating a whole fruit with it. Milk, cottage cheese, and eggs are also good sources of protein, as are bran muffins and whole wheat toast with peanut butter. But a word about the peanut butter you use.

Old-fashioned peanut butter, without preservatives (you keep it in the refrigerator after you have opened it) and with oil you have to mix in, is an excellent protein food. Hydrogenated peanut butter usually has sugar added and the hydrogenation process has turned the liquid oil into a solid fat. It has also turned unsaturated fatty acids into saturated ones. Now read the next guideline.

4. *Remember unsaturated fats are better than saturated fats.* In general, unsaturated fats are liquid at room temperature and saturated ones are solid. Most vegetable oils are unsaturated fats; the exceptions are coconut, palm, and cocoa. Saturated fats tend to increase cholesterol blood levels; mono-unsaturated fats (olive, avocado, and peanut oils) are neutral; and polyunsaturated fats (the rest of the vegetable oils) lower blood cholesterol levels. You should try to take twice as much unsaturated fat as saturated in your diet. (Remember, beef can be 50% to 75% saturated fat and only 25% protein.)

If you stop to read the labels on nondairy creamers (which many people use to avoid saturated fat), you'll see that most of them are made with coconut oil, a saturated fat. Half-and-half is better for you as far as your cholesterol level is concerned, because the nonfat part of milk contains a cholesterol-lowering factor.

Incidentally, new research has shown no direct correlation between cholesterol itself in the diet and blood levels of cholesterol. However, a diet high in saturated fats and cholesterol, in combination, may elevate cholesterol in the blood. Don't eat steak and eggs or bacon and eggs. Eat your eggs only with carbohydrates.

As I mentioned in relation to peanut butter, hydrogenation turns unsaturated oils into saturated fats as it solidifies them. One of the essential fatty acids, linoleic, is destroyed in the process. The fats that resulted from this alteration are unnatural "trans-fats," some of which have been linked to atherosclerosis and cancer. Until we know more about the long-term effects of these altered fats, it is probably best to avoid them; certainly, don't feed them to children.

5. *Use a variety of foods.* You should eat at least one food each day from each of the four food groups—whole grains; fruits and vegetables; milk and dairy products; fish, poultry, and meats. This way you are more likely to get all the essential nutrients you need in your diet. Let me focus on one example: Most adults don't drink enough milk or eat enough cheese. These foods are the main source of calcium. New research suggests you need about 1,000 milligrams (mg) of calcium in your diet each day to prevent the osteoporosis (bone softening) of old age. Your bones turn over their cells about every four months and, although they don't increase in size, they are still growing. The belief that you don't need calcium after you reach your grown height is totally wrong.

You need calcium for other purposes than making your bones hard. (And it is not calcium that makes arteries "hard"—that is cholesterol.) Calcium is necessary for the normal functioning of your nerves, contraction of your muscles, clotting of your blood, normal beating of your heart, and internal respiration of your cells.

Strange as it may seem, it is a lack of calcium in the diet rather than too much that causes the calcium deposits in the joints of elderly people. When calcium intake is low, the blood calcium level tends to lower, and this triggers the parathyroid gland to secrete a hormone that mobilizes calcium from the bones to maintain the correct level in the blood. It is this mobilized calcium that is deposited in the joints, not the dietary calcium. Excess dietary calcium either is not absorbed or is stored in the bones. Adequate dietary calcium intake "turns off" the parathyroid hormone.

An intake of 1,000 mg per day of calcium has also been shown to lower serum cholesterol levels and aid in the prevention of heart disease. One good way to get this amount of calcium is to drink a quart of skim milk every day. Milk is not just for kids anymore.

6. *Remember complex carbohydrates are better than sugars.* Most sugars

in processed food and table sugar are highly refined. They provide empty calories; that is, they add to our total calorie intake but supply no nutrients. The same thing can be said for alcohol—and it has twice the calories. Fruits and vegetables, especially starches, take longer to digest; they provide fiber, minerals, and vitamins, and are not likely to cause hypoglycemia. We must destroy the myth that starchy foods are fattening. Any food is fattening if taken in excess. Starches provide less than half (four calories per gram) the calories of fat (nine calories per gram) and fatty foods like beefsteak.

7. *Be aware that the ideal diet contains 58% carbohydrate, 12% protein, and 30% fat.* The carbohydrate should be made up of 40% to 45% complex carbohydrates (vegetables) and 15% sugars (orange juice). The fats should include twice as much unsaturated fat (20% vegetable oils) as saturated (10% animal fat). Training tables for athletes no longer promote steak and eggs; they now offer spaghetti and tomato sauce.

8. *Get as much of the protein as possible from vegetable sources.* Mexican children have blood cholesterol levels only half as high as white American children because their protein source is beans instead of meat. All legumes, especially soybeans and peanuts, are excellent sources. Animal sources of protein should favor fish over poultry, and poultry over meat. If you must eat meat, veal is preferred; then pork, lamb, and beef, in that order.

9. *As an adult, avoid vitamin supplements containing A and D.* Fortified milk supplies enough vitamin D and carrots are an adequate source of vitamin A. Supplements of these vitamins can be harmful over a long time period. (However, if you have just given up smoking, supplement your diet with 400 mg of vitamin E and 10 mg of vitamin A; it will help to restore the lining cells of your lungs.)

10. *Do not add salt to your food.* The average American gets too much salt. There is an adequate amount of salt in natural foods. Adding salt is just a bad habit that needs to be broken.

If you follow these guidelines, you probably will never have to worry about excess weight—as long as you also get adequate exercise.

Stress Management

Stress management depends on the acquisition of several learned skills. Hans Selye, who developed the concept of stress/distress, contended that stress can be good for us as well as bad. A stress-free environment would be intolerable. We need stress in order to live. Good stress produces the optimal level of stimulation for the individual to be productive and creative. Distress, however, is nonproductive, and we have to develop skills to deal with it.

There are two ways of dealing with distress. We can identify those things in our daily lives that cause distress and then design them out of our space. Or we can train ourselves to deal with the distress we can't avoid.

Dealing with stress can be likened to riding a wave on a surfboard. If you hit the wave right, you go faster and farther. If you hit it wrong, it can kill you. Therefore, it is essential that you learn how to ride with it.

Some of the learnable skills are relaxation techniques, assertiveness training, meditation, or human-potential-enhancing methods such as transactional analysis.

Physical Fitness

Physical fitness is the dimension of wellness that seems to enhance all the others. Regular exercise should become part of our lives. Preferably, it should be something we enjoy doing, something that is fun. Walking is probably the best exercise. It is something we can do all our lives, it can take us into beautiful surroundings, and we are all good at it.

Aerobic exercise consists of sustained physical activity for at least twelve to twenty minutes at a time. It improves oxygen use by our body and can be very helpful in preventing cardiovascular disease if performed three or four times a week. Examples are walking briskly, jogging, swimming, bicycling, cross-country skiing, and aerobic dance. (Sexual intercourse has also been known to qualify.)

Jogging has recently been downplayed. We are beginning to see too many bad side effects: shin splints, broken metatarsal bones in the foot, fallen arches, arthritis, menstrual disorders, and infertility in women. I personally believe it should be avoided by the nonathlete.

For the nonathlete who has not been exercising, it is important to begin slowly and cautiously with any marked increase in physical activity. Walking, again, is probably the safest way to start. The Canadian Air Force book on exercise offers graded programs based on age and sex differences to attain general body toning; this is an alternative way to begin.

Environmental Sensitivity

Environmental sensitivity is the fifth dimension of wellness. As Americans, we live in a relatively safe environment. However, as I pointed out earlier, new chemicals are being added to our environment at the rate of a thousand a year. The effects of these and the products of combustion on our air, water, and food chain should concern us all. As individuals, however, we can do little to change these except through the democratic process and making our concerns known. It is our immediate environments that require our personal, day-to-day attention.

Most of us are unaware that we can change our immediate environment almost at will. Even if we are aware that we are shaped and conditioned by this environment, we give little thought to changing it to work for us. Yet there is a lot at stake. If our environment is good, we will have increased energy and be able to grow. If it is bad, our energy decreases and we become bored with our life. The physiological effects of boredom are the same as those of stress; they can kill.

Obviously, we should eliminate anything around us that interferes with our achieving our potential and then restructure our space to enhance our well-being and self-actualization. Our space must match our values. Believing one thing and having to do another only leads to guilt and stress. Our space, our immediate environment, must become an extension of ourselves.

This aspect of wellness requires lifework planning. We should be able to write several scenarios for our life and choose the one that fits us best. We don't have to rely on chance and fate. We can become whatever we want to be. We should frequently ask ourselves: "If I were independently wealthy, would I be doing what I am doing today?" If not, then not being wealthy is no excuse.

Another approach is to write our own obituary. What would I want them to say about me? Which I do I want to be? This approach puts things in proper perspective. It forces us to face our own mortality, which in turn frees us to live up to our potential.

These are the five dimensions of wellness. If we put these elements into practice, if they govern our lifestyle, then we will have eliminated—without consciously planning to—the risk factors for all the leading causes of death. We can, of course, address each risk factor independently, in a piecemeal fashion. We will prevent disease, but we may not reach our optimal level of wellness.

On the other hand, practicing the dimensions of wellness—self-responsibility, nutritional awareness, stress management, physical fitness, and environmental sensitivity—offers a way of life that will be new to most of us. It is not easy to attain, but for those who have, it has been worth the effort. And it can offer each of us the opportunity for the first time to feel truly alive, to know what it means to be really healthy.

CHAPTER 26

A Letter to
Your Physician

Dear Colleagues:

This book is written as much for you as it is for the American public. Perhaps, because it is directed to your patients, you will be more likely to read it. I recall that when I was in private practice I regularly received an unsolicited journal listing "what your patients are reading." I made a point of always reading those articles in addition to the medical journals. If this service is no longer in operation, perhaps your patients will recommend you read at least this chapter. I welcome the opportunity to speak directly to you.

I love our profession, which is why events of the past ten years have disturbed me so. I have observed a growing disenchantment with our profession on the part of those we have dedicated our lives to serve. The miraculous breakthroughs in medical knowledge and technology during the 1950s and 1960s kept the public in awe of our potential power. We basked in their devotion and assured them there was no problem our technology could not solve. "Eat, drink, and be merry," we implied. "If tomorrow you become ill, we will save you."

We conquered infectious diseases, only to have them replaced with chronic diseases that we assume would fall equally well before our superior technology and knowledge. But we don't know how to cure atherosclerotic heart disease, or stroke, or cancer, or cirrhosis, or diabetes. And we don't understand the fundamental causes of these diseases.

We haven't lost our faith in technology; our love affair continues. Our patients, however, are beginning to have second thoughts about our magic powers. Some of you may not have noticed because you have been caught up, as I once was, in day-to-day practice. I realize how easy it is to be unaware of the larger picture when one is so busy with detail.

While we were not paying attention, a new epidemiological revolution took place. We are now in control of the infectious diseases. At present, chronic diseases are epidemic, although we may have difficulty associating their long, slow onset with an epidemic. Heart disease, cancer, and stroke are just as deadly as bubonic plague, yellow fever, and tuberculosis, and they are more prevalent and common among people today.

It is probably because of their slow onset and chronicity that epidemiology has become so important in their control and, therefore, to the practice of medicine. *The new knowledge provided by epidemiologists of the ten leading causes of death in the United States should be revolutionizing the practice of medicine.*

But it is not. It isn't that we have kept our heads in the sand; rather, they're in the clouds—that love affair is to blame. But let's not go into that . . . just yet. Let me tell you what I think we have missed.

Epidemiologists, working with a few of our colleagues, particularly cardiologists, have identified risk factors for these new epidemic diseases. Risk factors are elements that increase the probability of an individual's contracting a specific disease, and they can be identified in the individual beforehand, sometimes years before the onset of a disease. The longitudinal study of heart disease carried out in Framingham, Massachusetts, has contributed more than any other research to the identification of the risk factors for atherosclerotic heart disease.

Risk factors may simply be unhealthy behaviors (cigarette smoking is a good example). Or they may be bodily changes—signs, as we call them— that are measurable precursors of an actual disease (such as elevated serum cholesterol or high blood pressure).

All of us have had a great deal of experience searching for signs of disease. It is what we do each time we perform an annual physical exam— we look for signs of asymptomatic disease. But we are not accustomed to looking for behavioral risk factors or doing much about them, even if they are obvious.

What we have become really good at is establishing that a patient actually has a disease before it becomes symptomatic—for those few diseases that have an asymptomatic phase. But we are not used to identifying risk factors for a disease before its onset. Nor have we been taught how to help a patient eliminate a risk factor and prevent the onset of that disease.

We tell patients to stop smoking, lose weight, and get more exercise, but we don't have the skills necessary to really show them how to do it. We rely on their willpower and our authority and think that our responsibility is over—even when we know (now be honest) that they will not or cannot change. (As a matter of fact, we're not too good at changing our own behavior. As a profession, we have more drug addicts and suicides than most.)

Although we may believe that people really should quit smoking, lose weight, and get more exercise on general principles, we have never had any real evidence to push these changes. But now epidemiologists have shown that these behavioral risk factors are just as significant, if not more so, than the bodily changes that are prodromal of disease.

Actually, they are more important. They initiate the progression of events leading to the bodily changes. Moreover, since they precede these changes (by years sometimes), they are more amenable to reversal. It is correction in this area that is most likely to prevent disease.

And behavioral risk factors *can* be changed (see Chapter 24). As Dr. John Fahrquar, director of the Stanford Heart Disease Prevention Program, points out, we can prevent 90% of atherosclerotic heart disease and stroke just by eliminating three risk factors: cigarette smoking, high blood pressure, and elevated serum cholesterol. Similarly, 90% of lung cancer can be prevented if we help patients cut out cigarette smoking. These three diseases are the top three causes of death in the United States, accounting for 70% of all deaths. Just think: 90% *of the deaths from these diseases could be prevented by risk factor intervention, if it occurs early enough.*

In fact, 50% of all disease today could be prevented. Why aren't we willing to admit this? We continue to preoccupy ourselves with treating disease *after* it has occurred. Why don't we give equal consideration to prevention, let alone promotion of health? People are beginning to believe it is because we have a financial stake in their being sick. Is it?

There is a folk legend being told about our profession by epidemiologists and a growing number of knowledgeable consumers of health care— including some of your patients. We physicians are being likened to a tribe of healers whose praises were sung from coast to coast for their devotion to serving other people. It seems this tribe lived beside a raging white water river. Every year the tribe members saved more and more people from the waters. In fact, they were so busy rescuing people that they failed to question why these people had fallen into the river in the first place.

It seems that just a mile upstream, there was a bridge in such poor condition that people were falling into the river whenever they crossed the bridge. One day a wise man came along and noted the situation. "If you repair the bridge," he said to them, "people will not fall into the water."

"But we have been trained to pull people from the water," they replied. "It is not our job to prevent them from falling in."

* * *

Our neglect of prevention is not the only concern. The quality of our medical care is also being questioned. No one doubts that we can give the best medical care in the world. But we are beginning to coast on our laurels. I myself have been intimately associated with measuring the quality of medical care; I have written two texts on quality assurance and have watched the day-to-day delivery of care as the medical director of a large teaching hospital and as a board member of a foundation for medical care, a Professional Standards Review Organization. There is a lot of room for improvement. Our best is not good enough; we are not performing up to our potential.

Paradoxically, we are often providing too much care. Specialists make up 80% of our profession; only 20% of us are generalists. The opposite proportion is needed. In most cases, an individual seeking the services of a physician encounters someone who is overqualified to meet his or her needs. Consequently, most patients receive poor quality care at too high a price.

Most primary care in the United States today is provided by internists who expect their earnings to be commensurate with their board certification. It's not that the charges are out of proportion to the services rendered, but in most instances these services are more than are needed or necessary. This situation, I believe, is a main cause of the escalation in medical care costs—costs that reflect not only the high fee of a specialist but also the price of all the ancillary services the specialist orders.

Most internists are disease- and organ-system oriented. Look at the subspecialists in this field—allergists, barologists, cardiologists, dermatologists, endocrinologists, and so on—nearly one for every letter of the alphabet. What we need are more people-oriented physicians, especially in primary care. At present the people-oriented new specialty of family medicine numbers only 14.5% of all practicing physicians. By 1990, if our educational system doesn't change, their number will drop to 12.5%.

In the early 1970s, we cut out the rotating internship from our graduate medical education programs to permit specialization earlier in a physician's training. Even as I write this letter, I find an article in the *New England Journal of Medicine* that questions the wisdom of this move. Dr. Joseph Gonnella, director of medical education at Jefferson Medical College in Philadelphia, looks at "The Impact of Early Specialization on the Clinical Competence of Residents." He ends with a plea for "medical educators [to] restructure their programs to provide all physicians with a greater capacity to recognize the manifold nature of disease and trauma, and to provide more comprehensive care in the management of patients."*

* Joseph Gonnella, "The Impact of Early Specialization on the Clinical Competence of Residents."

The serious problem of overspecialization can be changed only by changing our medical education system, and only the profession can do that. There is a ten-year lag between changes made in the numbers and types of physicians we educate and the finished product, the practicing physician. Read the report of the Graduate Medical Education National Advisory Committee, discussed in Chapter 13. It predicts that by 1990 we will have a surplus of 70,000 physicians, most of them specialists. We will be compounding the mismatch between the medical needs of the American people and the configuration of the profession.

Our knowledge and its associated technology can now provide much more care than the public needs. I'm not suggesting we move backward. We should retain our present capabilities. But we do not need all the specialists we are training to do this. Unless we change the proportions, our care will be more related to what we know than to what people need.

We have created a Medical Establishment that I have likened to a dinosaur. It has outgrown its usefulness and ability to survive. Daily, it demands more fodder for its technology, more people to fill its hospital beds and operating suites, more cases to pay for its capability in sophisticated ancillary services, its space age laboratories and X-ray departments and the technicians who staff them. In short, the Medical Establishment is too big and too costly. It is driving us into bankruptcy.

As physicians, we have been taught that if there is anything we can do for a patient, it is our moral obligation to give him or her the advantage of at least a trial treatment to see if it works. Today, however, we are faced with an almost unlimited storehouse of possible treatments and the stock of new miracle drugs and techniques keeps growing. We are very close to the point where we will cease to serve the best interests of our patients. We could easily step over the line and begin to use our patients for our own ends. Many believe we are already there.

The American public is beginning to question our motivations. Government and business are asking why health care expenditures are increasing at three times the rate of the gross national product. The 1982 increase of 17.5% in hospital costs was nearly three times the rate of increase in the Consumer Price Index. Physicians' fees also exceeded the CPI by several percentage points. Physicians' income has increased 100% in the last ten years. (Today the average physician nets $70,000 from an annual business grossing $120,000.) Physicians, moreover, generate 85% of hospital costs by controlling who is hospitalized, how long they stay, what tests are ordered, and what services are offered by the institution.

We continue to act as if our health resources were infinite. (I spoke of this in detail in Chapter 9, in portraying the tragedy of the medical commons.) We act as if no one cared how much we spend on medical care. As if whatever we deemed necessary would be acceptable.

Nothing could be further from the truth. If you have not heard the cry for cost containment coming from the public and government, you will soon hear it loud and clear from American business.

The Washington (D.C.) Business Group on Health, composed of many of the Fortune 500 companies, was formed a few years ago, primarily to contain health care costs. There are now sixty to seventy of these coalitions throughout the United States, in every city with a major business complex. They have banded together to fight.

Employers are the largest purchasers of health care, in the form of benefits for their employees and their employees' dependents. The cost of the same benefit package has been increasing at a rate of 15% to 30% a year, and employers are naturally concerned. Moreover, payroll taxes have increased because employers are paying half the cost of Medicare and Medicaid.

The message is loud and clear—our health resources are finite. We have reached the limit to which business is willing to go without demanding a reorganization of our delivery system. They are already looking at the alternatives, at health maintenance organizations and independent practice associations. It could be only a short step to excluding all payment to practitioners who do not prospectively contract with industry to provide care for their employees at a negotiated, but fixed, rate.

The business coalitions are also embracing disease prevention and health promotion programs in the workplace. Over 400 companies have started fitness programs, and they are expanding into more comprehensive programs of health promotion. Risk factor intervention is a strategy for cost containment that business could implement *outside* the Medical Establishment.

The handwriting is on the wall. The Medical Establishment could become a second Detroit. We are all familiar with the devastating effect on the American auto industry when consumers refused to buy its product and turned to foreign imports that more closely met their needs for compact economy cars with high gas mileage. Our profession is in the same position Detroit was in a few years ago. The public may soon refuse to buy our chrome-plated, high-technology, high-cost impersonal health care, and may turn somewhere else.

Where will they turn? A burgeoning flea market of alternative health care providers is standing in the wings, waiting for the medical profession to do itself in by worshiping the golden calf. You may feel safe because you think all the kooks and cults are in California. But think a moment.

In the recent past, what started in California in health care innovation was often adopted by the rest of the country in less than five years. Remember group practice, peer review, foundations for medical care, utilization review, HMOs, emergency medical services, advertising by physicians? They all started in California and moved east.

The American public became interested in healthy lifestyles and the promotion of wellness in the 1960s. Most of our profession ignored this. The joggers, health food stores, fitness programs, health spas—we thought they were a passing fad, soon to be relegated to the same closet as the hula hoop. But these "fads" are still with us, and they're growing stronger.

What we didn't anticipate—and still don't believe—is that these "health freaks" could inadvertently eliminate most of the risk factors for atherosclerotic heart disease and cause its incidence to decrease 22% from 1968 to 1978, *without any intervention or help from the medical profession.*

Epidemiologists realize it. Public health physicians realize it. Government, business, and the general public have come to realize it. Only the medical profession has failed to realize the reason for it. All we do is clap ourselves on the back and take credit for it—if it has to do with disease, it must be something we did, even if we don't know what.

Half of our present disease will be prevented in the next ten years with or without the help of the medical profession. I, for one, hope it occurs within the profession. The practice of medicine is not just the diagnosis and treatment of disease but also the restoration and preservation of health.

Many will say we must first understand the cause of a disease before we can prevent it. This is only partially true. We certainly do not know all there is to know about the causes of the diseases that are epidemic today. But epidemiologists have shown us their natural history and identified risk factors related to their cause. If Jenner had the courage to begin his inoculations to prevent smallpox 150 years before we knew it was caused by a virus, then we certainly should have the courage to begin to prevent diseases in our time by risk factor intervention.

We have eliminated smallpox without ever discovering how to cure it. Perhaps we can do the same for atherosclerotic heart disease, stroke, and lung cancer.

As I tried to point out in Chapters 24 and 25, disease prevention by risk factor intervention and health promotion to prevent the development of the risk factors in the first place are both aspects of the same concept; only the approach is different. And it is this concept that I believe will dominate health care in our time.

Risk factor identification and elimination must become a routine part of periodic health evaluations within the practice of medicine. Unless we want to lose our autonomy and wind up as only a small component of the entire health picture, we must begin to modify our own behavior.

We, too, must reclaim our life—our profession. We must reclaim that part of the practice of medicine we have neglected—the restoration and preservation of health. To succeed, we must do several things:

1. We must take responsibility for our own profession and rededicate our lives to serve the medical and health care needs of the American people.

2. We must realign the numbers, types, and distribution of physicians to match the public's needs. This will require a sharp reduction in the number of physicians we train in the various specialties, with a marked increase in the number of family practice physicians. As a goal for 1990, we should aim for 50% family practitioners, 17% specialists who provide some primary care (general internists, pediatricians, and obstetricians), and 33% specialists who provide secondary and tertiary care.

3. We must recognize that our nation's health care resources are finite and, as a profession, we must exercise mutual coercion to preserve the medical commons (reread Chapter 9).

4. We must embrace the concept of risk factor intervention as the key to disease prevention and incorporate the identification of risk factors as part of a lifetime health-monitoring program for our patients.

5. We must acquire the skills in behavioral change necessary to help our patients, our clients, prevent disease.

6. We must reclaim our own lives so we may serve as role models for those we have dedicated our lives to serve.

A Matter of Life and Death: Reprise

I HAVE often wondered how my life might have been different had I changed just one event, taken a different path somewhere along the way. What if I had joined the navy instead of the army? I wouldn't have been stationed on Governor's Island, where I met my wife. But would I have met her anyway, somewhere else—so that the choice would have amounted to only a short detour instead of a totally different life? I'm afraid I don't believe in predestination as my Presbyterian parents did. I'm glad I chose the army; I don't want to think about a life without Sandy or even to contemplate that our two children might never have existed. It is too frightening.

But that is what I am about to do in the life of Adam Americus. I'm going to change one event. In his case—and I believe the same would be true in ours—from that point on, his life was totally different. Let's start again at the beginning.

You remember Adam Americus. He was born in 1930, a child of the Depression, a teenager during World War II, an all-American football player in college. After two years in Korea, he takes off his uniform and easily slips into the male harness. He marries his childhood sweetheart and becomes a father and an M.B.A. a year later. He joins one of the big eight accounting firms and learns how to work under pressure and deadlines, solving other people's problems.

Adam seems to thrive on the competition; he fights his way rapidly from consultant to manager to partner in five years. After three more children at two-year intervals, he has a vasectomy on the advice of his wife's obstetrician. But an affair with his secretary cinches his harness even tighter. As penance, he works harder and starts going to church every Sunday. He eats more, smokes more, drinks more. The competition is getting tougher, and his indigestion more frequent. He is buying Tums by the gross.

It's time for his annual physical, which his firm insists upon. Adam approaches this ritual with his typical macho bravado. He won't admit to any real symptoms. And he gets the same advice he always has from the doctor the company sends him to. "Your blood pressure is a little high and your cholesterol is up a bit. You should take more time off, relax more, lose some weight, and cut down on your smoking," intones the doctor, as he pats his own paunch and blows smoke in Adam's face.

But now it is 1970. Adam is again going for his annual physical. He is in for a surprise—a change has been made. The doctor with the paunch, the one who blew smoke in Adam's face, died of a coronary. He has been replaced by Jon Smith, M.D., one of the new specialists in family practice.

On his first visit, Adam fills out an eight-page questionnaire and then goes through what the nurse calls multiphasic health testing. Now he has come to see the doctor.

"Sorry to hear about the old doc," begins Adam. This one looks more like a jock than a doc, he thinks to himself.

"Apparently he died very suddenly. His partner asked me to take his place. I just finished my training and passed my boards."

"Oh, so you are a specialist?" Adam remarks.

"Yes, it's a new specialty—family practice."

"Like a general practitioner?"

"No, not quite. We both practice primary care but family physicians have more training—four years of residency. It's a new kind of specialty, a specialty in treating families. Family physicians are the doctors you first contact when you get sick, but we are more concerned about keeping you healthy. We like to have a long-term contract with you for your family's health care needs—not a contract in writing, but an understanding."

"A family doctor?" Adam reflects. "Can't believe it. We sure need one. I've got four kids. My wife will certainly dig you."

"Well, my job is to keep her digging you," Dr. Smith joshes him. "And to keep you from digging your grave."

"What? My grave? What are you talking about, Doc? Is something wrong with me?"

"Call me Jon, if you don't mind. May I call you Adam?"

"Sure, but what did you find?"

"No disease, Adam. Not yet. But you are well on your way to developing heart disease."

"Heart disease? But I've never had any trouble with my heart. Damn it. I played football, you know."

"Remember that questionnaire you filled out for me last week? It's what we call a Health Hazard Appraisal. You might have noticed there were a lot of questions about your lifestyle."

"Yes, I remember. It sure sounded dumb. What difference does it make how many miles I drive on a fucking highway? Or how often I wear a seat belt? Who the hell cares?"

"That wasn't the significant part for you, Adam. But several other questions were very important. Your main health hazard is that you smoke. And you're a heavy smoker—three packs a day. You're also twenty pounds overweight, and you don't get much exercise. It's obvious you eat the wrong foods—your cholesterol is 285. And what about your job? Is it very stressful? Something seems to be getting to you—your blood pressure is 185/95, much too high."

"Come on, Doc—I mean, Jon. Why sound so serious? They've been telling me that for years. You haven't even examined me and you practically have me in my grave."

"The Health Hazard Appraisal and those tests you had last week have given me more information about you than I could possibly get from examining you. But we'll get around to that today. I do want to confirm some of the findings. Isn't what I have been telling you about your habits correct?"

"Yes, it's true, but so what? I've tried to stop smoking, but it made me uptight. Started yelling at Alice and the kids. And if I cut out cigarettes, I gain weight. I quit for ten days once and gained ten pounds. And I can't do anything about my job, you know. I've got a family to worry about."

"Yes, Adam, you do have to worry about your family. Your life insurance can't replace you."

"Come on, Jon, you're scaring the hell out of me."

"I mean to, Adam. Your life is in danger. But it's not all bad news. If you are willing to work at it, you can prevent a heart attack. Those findings I told you about are what we call risk factors. It means there's a high probability that you will have a coronary heart attack within five to ten years—if you don't change the way you live and break some of your bad habits.

"Let me tell you about a study they did in Framingham, Massachusetts. They were interested in the natural history of atherosclerotic heart disease—that's another name for a coronary. I trained in New England, so I got some inside information on the probabilities they worked out for developing the disease. It depends on the number of risk factors an individual has working against him. You have several.

I calculated your Framingham Risk Score last night, Adam, based on your test findings. It was 543. That means you have a 54.3% probability of developing a coronary in eight years. That's more than even money, if you're a betting man."

"How can you be so sure?"

"I can't be positive. But those were the probabilities for forty-five-year-old men in Framingham with the same risk factors you have: cholesterol 285, blood pressure 185/95, heavy smoking. Also, your EKG showed some beginning left ventricular hypertrophy—that means your heart is reacting to the strain you have put it under.

"Besides, you have a family history of heart disease. Your father and your grandfather before him—both had coronaries at an early age. I can't change your parents. That's a biological risk factor. But together we can change the others."

"Okay, Jon, you've convinced me. How do we begin? And when?"

They begin that very day. With Jon's help, Adam enrolls in a smoking cessation program and quits five weeks later. He has never smoked again.

Jon puts him on a 2,000-calorie diet and educates him and his wife, Alice, about eating correctly. Adam's fat intake is restricted to only 10% of his total calories; it is all poly- and mono-unsaturated, no saturated fats. He gets 12% protein, mostly from vegetable sources; the rest is carbohydrate, 15% sugar and 63% complex carbohydrates. To Adam's surprise, he learns that starch isn't fattening. Spaghetti and tomato sauce with soybean balls fill him up.

Adam also starts doing aerobic exercise, beginning with brisk walking and then tennis. Through it all, Adam and Jon become great friends. They're playing tennis together now, three days a week.

Another change comes from Jon's suggestion that Adam take a course in transcendental meditation and another on time management. Adam gets so much out of them that on his own he enrolls in a transactional analysis program and an assertiveness training class.

In 1975, Adam is asked to become president of a small electronics firm in town. He's quite happy with his new job. Although he still encounters stress, he knows how to deal with it—to his advantage.

At his most recent periodic health evaluation, in 1982, Adam's cholesterol was 175; his blood pressure, 140/80; and his EKG, normal. He is fit and trim, in tune with his body. He could almost be playing football again in college. Even his sex life has improved. "It's good I had that vas ligation so many years ago," he tells Jon with a laugh.

Adam's Framingham Risk Score is now 35—only a 3.5% probability of developing a coronary. "Go ahead," says Jon. "Live it up, have fun, be happy."

At fifty-one, Adam Americus has succeeded. He has reclaimed his own life and knows what it means to be healthy. He's going strong. That one event—it really was a matter of life or death. ❧

APPENDIX I

Smoking Cessation Program

THIS PROGRAM is based on one advocated by the U.S. Department of Health and Human Services in a booklet entitled *Calling it Quits; The Latest Advice on How to Give Up Cigarettes.* I have augmented the program and changed the format according to my own experience as I stopped smoking, but if any part of it does not fit your personality or beliefs, then change that part to fit *you.*

Week 1

GOAL   To learn everything you need to know about cigarette smoking and how it affects your health.

REFERENCE TEXT   *The Smoking Digest,* available from the Office of Cancer Communications, National Cancer Institute, Building 31, Room 10 A 16, Bethesda, Md. 20014

ACTIVITIES

- Read text.
- Visit and pick up literature from the local offices of the American Cancer Society (literature on lung cancer), American Heart Association (smoking and heart disease), American Lung Association (emphysema and chronic obstructive lung disease).
- Try to find someone to quit with you; two or three are even better. Be sure to include your spouse if he or she smokes. But don't put it off if you can't find anyone else; you *can* do it alone.

Week 2

GOAL   To realize you *can* quit! (You may not *want* to yet but by now you should realize that you *should.* Thirty million Americans have already quit. You can be number 30,000,001.)

ACTIVITIES

- List all the reasons you want to quit.
- Every night before you go to bed, repeat a different one of the reasons, out loud, ten times.
- Meet once this week with those who are going to quit with you. Set a date to meet each week. Compare your lists of reasons to quit. Also *set a date when you will all quit* sometime during the fifth week. (Once this date is set do not change it!)
- Calculate how much you spent on cigarettes last year. Outline what you are going to do with the money this next year.
- Stop buying cigarettes by the carton. Switch brands among those with the same nicotine content. Do not smoke two packs of the same brand in a row.
- Begin walking two half-miles each day.
- Get eight hours' sleep each night.
- Drink three glasses of water each day, with meals.
- Call your dentist and make an appointment to have your teeth cleaned on the day you will quit.

Week 3

GOAL To cut your smoking in half.

ACTIVITIES

- Continue with all activities from Week 2.
- Keep track of each cigarette you smoke this week. To do this, wrap a piece of blank paper around your pack of cigarettes and hold it with a rubber band.
- On the *first day*, write down the time you smoke each cigarette. Place an asterisk after the time if you smoke that cigarette within thirty minutes of getting up, going to bed, having sex, after a meal, or if you have it with coffee or alcohol or while you are driving.
- At the *end of the first day*, examine your smoking patterns and associations by observing the asterisks on your score card.
- On the *second day*, eliminate half of the cigarettes you smoked at the times marked by the asterisks.
- On the *third day*, eliminate the cigarettes marked by the remaining asterisks. This means that from now on you will not smoke while driving, drinking coffee or alcohol, or within thirty minutes of getting up, going to bed, or after meals. (I tried rewarding myself by forgetting about the ones associated with sex.)
- Begin brushing your teeth immediately after every meal if you aren't already doing this.
- On the *fourth day*, switch to cigarette brands with only half the nicotine content of your usual brand.
- Increase your water intake to six glasses a day. (And don't smoke when you get up at night to urinate.)

- Don't keep your cigarettes in your pocket or purse from now on. Keep them out of sight or easy reach in a drawer at home and at the office.
- Increase your walking to one mile each day. Breathe deeply several times during the walk and do not smoke. (Doesn't the clean air feel good in your lungs?)

Week 4

GOAL   To eliminate the remaining nicotine from your system.

ACTIVITIES

- Continue all activities from Week 3.
- Switch to the two brands with the lowest nicotine content you can find. Alternate packs.
- Increase the interval of not smoking to one hour after getting up, before going to bed, and after meals.
- When you crave a cigarette, don't smoke. Instead, act out the lighting and smoking of an imaginary cigarette. Inhale slowly and deeply for two minutes. Now, if you still want a cigarette, go ahead.
- Smoke only when you really want a cigarette. If you don't smoke, reward yourself with a stick of sugar-free gum.
- Put all the butts from the cigarettes you smoke this week into a large glass jar, one-quarter full of water. Look at the jar and smell it just before you eat.
- Plan how you are going to reward yourself on the day you will quit. (Remember you have all that money you are going to save next year.)

Week 5

GOAL   To smoke your last cigarette.

ACTIVITIES

- Continue all activities from Week 4 up until the day you quit.
- On the night before you will quit, smoke your last cigarette. Flush *all* remaining cigarettes in the house down the toilet, including the jar of butts you've been saving. Hide all lighters and ashtrays.
- On the first day of the rest of your life, call the friends in your group and congratulate them on quitting.
- Go have your teeth cleaned.
- Keep busy. Maybe take in a movie.
- Reward yourself with the special celebration you have planned.
- Keep drinking six glasses of water a day for the next three days.
- Brush your teeth after every meal and as often as you want.
- Meet with your group the day after you quit. Again, congratulate each other. Look at some cigarette advertisements and notice what they have been trying to do to you. Laugh about it. Write a group letter to the tobacco company. (You don't have to mail it.)

- If you crave a cigarette, smoke an imaginary one for three minutes. The craving will go away. But if it is still there, call someone in your group and talk about it. But don't smoke.

Weeks 6, 7, 8

GOAL To not start smoking again and to reorganize your life as a non-smoker.

ACTIVITIES

- Continue to meet with your group at least once a week. Talk on the phone several times.
- Keep brushing your teeth after every meal.
- If you need something to do with your hands, play with something, like a pencil.
- If you miss having something in your mouth, smoke that imaginary cigarette, use a toothpick, or chew a stick of sugarless gum. Try not to substitute snack foods. If you need to munch, use only celery or carrot sticks.
- Switch to decaffeinated coffee. It will lower your craving for a cigarette and decrease the heartburn you may be experiencing.
- Begin to associate with nonsmokers. (Aren't you glad your gang quit with you?)
- Spend more time in places that do not permit smoking.
- Switch to activities that would make smoking difficult: swimming, tennis, handball.
- Be particularly active with your hands. Try biking, crossword puzzles, needlework, painting. Do all the repairs you can think of around the house.
- Stretch a lot.
- Pay attention to your appearance. Replace any clothes that have cigarette burns on them.
- Plan a monthly celebration on the anniversary of your big day.

Congratulations! You are quite a person. Begin to love yourself more. You deserve it. You have accomplished one of the most difficult tasks a human being ever had to do. You have not only broken a bad habit but you have also overcome an addiction. Now that you realize you will never smoke another cigarette again as long as you live, *the craving will go away.* (But it will hang around until you realize this.)

Health Hazard Appraisal

The 4-page and 8-page questionnaires for the Health Hazard Appraisal that can be obtained from Medical Datamation are reprinted with their permission. In addition, sample reports to the individual are included. Actual questionnaires can be obtained by writing to the following address:

Medical Datamation
Bellevue, Ohio 44811

or by calling (800) 537-2893

SAMPLE 4-Page Questionnaire

Develops Lifestyle Index

and Health Risk Index

ur Facility Name
dress
ty, State
p

)TE: *Please follow directions carefully. If you consider a question too personal, you may skip it. All information will be handled confidentially.*

TIFICATION

Name |_|_|_|_|_|_|_|_|_|_|_|_|_|_|_|_|_|_|_|_|_|_|_|_|_|_|_|_|
Last Name, First Name, Middle Name

oday's Date |_|_|–|_|_|–|_|_| 12 Birth Date |_|_|–|_|_|–|_|_|
        Mo.   Da.   Yr.   *Mo.   Da.   Yr.*

ocial Security Number |_|_|_|–|_|_|–|_|_|_|_| 14 ○ None

○ Female   16 ○ Male

Height _____ ft. _____ in.   18 Weight _____ lbs.

MANENT HOME ADDRESS

treet |_|_|_|_|_|_|_|_|_|_|_|_|_|_|_|_|_|_|_|_|_|_|_|_|_|_|_|

City |_|_|_|_|_|_|_|_|_|_|_|_|_|_|_|_|_|_|_|_|_|_|_|_|_|_|_|

State or Province |_|_|_|_|_|_|_|_|_|_|_|_|_|_|_|_|_|_|_|_|_|

Zip |_|_|_|_|_|

Country |_|_|_|_|_|_|_|_|_|_|_|_|_|_|_|_|_|_|_|_|_|_|_|_|

1-604

DEMOGRAPHIC Background

Race

10 ○ American Indian
11 ○ Black
12 ○ Caucasian
13 ○ Other

Family income level

14 ○ Low
15 ○ Middle
16 ○ High

Marital Status

17 ○ Single
18 ○ Married
19 ○ Widowed
20 ○ Separated
21 ○ Divorced

ESSES and MEDICAL PROBLEMS

k the problems you have or have had that have been
nosed or treated by a physician or other health professional.

s	No	Problem		Yes	No	Problem
)	○	Alcoholism				High blood fats, specify.
)	○	Anemia-sickle cell	35	○	○	Cholesterol
)	○	Bleeding trait	36	○	○	Triglycerides
)	○	Bronchitis, chronic	37	○	○	High blood pressure
		Cancer	38	○	○	High blood pressure,
)	○	Breast				uncontrolled
)	○	Cervix	39	○	○	Obesity - more than
)	○	Colon				20 lbs. overweight
)	○	Lung	40	○	○	Pneumonia
)	○	Uterus	41	○	○	Polyps in colon
)	○	Other Cancer	42	○	○	Rheumatic fever
)	○	Cirrhosis - liver	43	○	○	Rheumatic fever, with
)	○	Colitis - ulcerative				resultant heart murmur
)	○	Depression	44	○	○	Stroke
)	○	Diabetes	45	○	○	Suicide attempt
)	○	Diabetes, uncontrolled	46	○	○	Tuberculosis
)	○	Emphysema		Yes	No	In the past year,
)	○	Fibrocystic breasts				have you had -
		Heart problem	47	○	○	Chest pain on exer-
)	○	Heart attack				tion relieved by rest?
)	○	Coronary disease	48	○	○	Shortness of breath
)	○	Rheumatic heart				lying down, relieved
)	○	Heart valve prob.				by sitting up?
)	○	Heart murmur	49	○	○	Unexplained weight
)	○	Enlarged heart				loss more than 10 lbs.
)	○	Heart rhythm prob.	50	○	○	Unexplained rectal
)	○	Other heart prob.				bleeding?
			51	○	○	Unexplained vaginal
						bleeding?

2-105

FEELINGS

Mark the frequency with which you have the feelings listed by
marking in the appropriate column.

M-Most of time   S-Some of time   R-Rarely or none

	M	S	R	
10	○	○	○	Feel sad, depressed?
11	○	○	○	Wish to end it all?
12	○	○	○	Feel tense and anxious?
13	○	○	○	Worry about things generally?
14	○	○	○	More aggressive, hard-driving than
				friends?
15	○	○	○	Have an intense desire to achieve?
16	○	○	○	Feel optimistic about the future?

FAMILY MEDICAL HISTORY (Blood Relatives)

Check items that apply for your blood relatives. **Your blood
relatives include your children, brothers, sisters, parents, and**
grandparents.

30 ○ Do not know my family medical history.

(Go to next section)

Yes	No	Illness		Yes	No	Illness
31	○	○	Anemia-sickle	36	○	○	High blood pressure
			cell	37	○	○	Mental illness
32	○	○	Bleeding trait	38	○	○	Stroke
33	○	○	Cancer	39	○	○	Suicide
34	○	○	Diabetes (sugar)	40	○	○	Tuberculosis
35	○	○	Heart disease				

Yes	No	Check the items that apply.
50 ○	○	Father died of a heart attack before age 60?
51 ○	○	Mother died of a heart attack before age 60?
52 ○	○	Mother or sister had cancer of the breast?
53 ○	○	Did your mother take DES (diethylstilbestrol)
		when she was pregnant with you?

41   1

HABITS and RISK FACTORS

Your habits influence your ability to achieve and maintain good health and long life.

EATING

Yes	No	Do you usually or generally-
10 ○	○	Consider yourself overweight?
11 ○	○	Follow a restricted diet for medical reasons?
12 ○	○	Eat 3 meals a day?
13 ○	○	Snack between meals?
14 ○	○	Know what foods are high in carbohydrates, starches?
15 ○	○	Know what foods are high in cholesterol?
16 ○	○	Know what foods are high in fiber?
17 ○	○	Know the difference between saturated and unsaturated fats?
18 ○	○	Know how to count calories accurately without the aid of a book?
19 ○	○	Eat fried foods 5 or more times per week?
20 ○	○	Eat "out" 5 or more times per week (food not cooked at home)?

Specify number of servings you eat during a typical DAY (24 hrs.)

DAILY BASIS-

Type of food	DON'T EAT	Usual servings per DAY- 1 or less 2 3 4 5 6 7 or more
31 Fruit or fruit juice	○	①②③④⑤⑥⑦
32 Vegetables	○	①②③④⑤⑥⑦
33 Cereal-non pre-sweetened	○	①②③④⑤⑥⑦
34 Bread, rolls, biscuits, bagels	○	①②③④⑤⑥⑦
35 White bread, rolls, biscuits	○	①②③④⑤⑥⑦
36 Potatoes, rice, macaroni, pastas	○	①②③④⑤⑥⑦
37 Pie, cake, doughnuts, sweet rolls	○	①②③④⑤⑥⑦
38 Meat or meat substitutes-beef, pork, cheese, poultry, fish	○	①②③④⑤⑥⑦
39 Soybeans, lentils, legumes, nuts, peanut butter	○	①②③④⑤⑥⑦
40 Skim milk	○	①②③④⑤⑥⑦
41 2% milk	○	①②③④⑤⑥⑦
42 Whole milk	○	①②③④⑤⑥⑦
43 Butter, margarine (tsp.)	○	①②③④⑤⑥⑦
44 Soft drinks (regular, non-diet)	○	①②③④⑤⑥⑦
45 Caffeinated coffee, tea, cola	○	①②③④⑤⑥⑦
46 Beer or wine	○	①②③④⑤⑥⑦
47 Salt (shaker use)	○	①②③④⑤⑥⑦
48 Pretzels, crackers	○	①②③④⑤⑥⑦
49 Potato or corn chips, french fries	○	①②③④⑤⑥⑦
50 Sugar (tsp.)	○	①②③④⑤⑥⑦

Specify number of servings you eat during a typical WEEK (7 days).
Keep in mind there are 21 meals/week.

WEEKLY BASIS

Type of Food	DON'T EAT	Usual servings per WEEK- 1 or less 2 3 4 5 6 7 or more
51 Beef or lamb	○	①②③④⑤⑥⑦
52 Pork, bacon, sausage	○	①②③④⑤⑥⑦
53 Weiners, lunchmeats	○	①②③④⑤⑥⑦
54 Poultry or fish	○	①②③④⑤⑥⑦
55 Shrimp, lobster, clams	○	①②③④⑤⑥⑦
56 Eggs	○	①②③④⑤⑥⑦
57 Hard cheese	○	①②③④⑤⑥⑦
58 Cottage cheese, soft cheese	○	①②③④⑤⑥⑦
59 Ice Cream, milk shakes	○	①②③④⑤⑥⑦
60 Salad oil, sour cream, mayonnaise	○	①②③④⑤⑥⑦
61 Candy	○	①②③④⑤⑥⑦

EXERCISE

Yes	No	Do you-
10 ○	○	Know the type of exercise that may help to prevent heart attacks?
11 ○	○	Know how to take your own pulse and monitor the effects of exercise?
12 ○	○	Get regular strenuous exercise, such as jogging, for at least 20 minutes 3 times a week?
13 ○	○	Get regular exercise of any type?

If "Yes" to item 13, complete the section below. If "No," go to item 40 below.

	Don't Do This	Frequency (DAYS per WEEK) 1 2 3 4 5 6 7	Length of each session (MINUTES per DAY) 10 20 30 40
14 Walking slow (20 min/mile)	○	①②③④⑤⑥⑦	⑩⑳㉚㊵
15 Walking fast (15 min/mile)	○	①②③④⑤⑥⑦	⑩⑳㉚㊵
16 Jogging (10 min/mile)	○	①②③④⑤⑥⑦	⑩⑳㉚㊵
17 Running (8 min/mile)	○	①②③④⑤⑥⑦	⑩⑳㉚㊵
18 Cycling slow (6 mph)	○	①②③④⑤⑥⑦	⑩⑳㉚㊵
19 Cycling fast (12 mph)	○	①②③④⑤⑥⑦	⑩⑳㉚㊵
20 Swimming slow (25 yds/min)	○	①②③④⑤⑥⑦	⑩⑳㉚㊵
21 Swimming fast (50 yds/min)	○	①②③④⑤⑥⑦	⑩⑳㉚㊵
Racquet sports			
22 Recreational or doubles	○	①②③④⑤⑥⑦	⑩⑳㉚㊵
23 Competitive or singles	○	①②③④⑤⑥⑦	⑩⑳㉚㊵
24 Calisthenics	○	①②③④⑤⑥⑦	⑩⑳㉚㊵
25 Dancing	○	①②③④⑤⑥⑦	⑩⑳㉚㊵
26 Basketball, football, soccer or similar sport	○	①②③④⑤⑥⑦	⑩⑳㉚㊵
27 Weight training	○	①②③④⑤⑥⑦	⑩⑳㉚㊵
28 Golf or bowling	○	①②③④⑤⑥⑦	⑩⑳㉚㊵
29 Downhill skiing in season	○	①②③④⑤⑥⑦	⑩⑳㉚㊵
30 Cross country skiing in season	○	①②③④⑤⑥⑦	⑩⑳㉚㊵

SMOKING

Yes	No	Do you-
40 ○	○	Smoke a pipe and inhale 5 or more times/day?
41 ○	○	Smoke cigars and inhale 5 or more times/day?
42 ○	○	Have you ever smoked cigarettes?

If so, specify amount and duration.

	Daily amount		Number of years
43 ○	1/2 pack/day or less	47 ○	Less than 1 year
44 ○	1/2 to 1 pack/day	48 ○	1 to 5 years
45 ○	1 to 2 packs/day	49 ○	5 to 10 years
46 ○	Over 2 packs/day	50 ○	Over 10 years

Yes	No	
51 ○	○	Do you currently smoke cigarettes?

If you used to smoke cigarettes, but stopped, specify number of years since you stopped.

52 ○ 1 yr.	55 ○ 4 yrs.	58 ○ 7 yrs.
53 ○ 2 yrs.	56 ○ 5 yrs.	59 ○ 8 yrs.
54 ○ 3 yrs.	57 ○ 6 yrs.	60 ○ 9 or more yrs.

HOL

No
- ○ Do you currently drink alcohol?
- ○ Did you formerly drink alcohol but stopped?

have ever drunk alcohol, specify details.

te the number of drinks consumed during a typical drinking
ion (a drink is a bottle of beer, a shot of whiskey, or equivalent).

1 to 2 drinks	14 ○	6 to 10 drinks
2 to 6 drinks	15 ○	Over 10 drinks

e average, indicate the amount and duration at this level.

Amount per week		Number of years
Less than 2 drinks/wk.	21 ○	Less than one year
2 to 10 drinks/wk.	22 ○	1 to 5 years
10 to 25 drinks/wk.	23 ○	5 to 10 years
25 to 40 drinks/wk.	24 ○	10 to 20 years
Over 40 drinks/wk.	25 ○	Over 20 years

3S

No Do you-
- ○ Know the short and long term effects of street drugs?
- ○ Have a problem with drugs?
- ○ Want help with drug counseling?

JMA, ACCIDENTS and OTHER HAZARDS

No Do you, or are you-
- ○ Frequently exposed to industrial chemicals?
- ○ Frequently exposed to insecticides and pesticides?
- ○ Exposed to loud noise without ear protection?
- ○ Operate or work around industrial or farm machinery?
- ○ Climb or work on ladders, scaffolds?
- ○ Water ski or boat without a life preserver?
- ○ Know how to swim?
- ○ Live in an area where violent crime is common?
- ○ Know how to give basic first aid, life support (CPR, cardiac resuscitation, mouth-to-mouth breathing)?
- ○ Drive after drinking alcohol or taking drugs?
- ○ Ride with drivers who have been drinking alcohol or taking drugs?
- ○ Tend to exceed the speed limit?

many miles do you travel in a car or other motor vehicle each
(average is 12,000 miles)?

○ Up to 10,000	44 ○	15,000 to 20,000
○ 10,000 to 15,000	45 ○	Over 20,000

t percent of the time do you wear a seat belt?

○ 0 to 25%	46 ○	50% to 75%
○ 25% to 50%	49 ○	75% to 100%

t percent of the time do you wear a shoulder strap?

○ 0 to 25%	52 ○	50 to 75%
○ 25% to 50%	53 ○	75% to 100%

STRESS

Specify CHANGES that have occurred in your life in the PAST YEAR.

10 ○	Spouse died	17 ○	Got divorced or separated
11 ○	Close family member died	18 ○	Lost a lot of money
12 ○	Moved to a new town	19 ○	Took on a lot of debt
13 ○	Changed jobs	20 ○	Got married
14 ○	Son/daughter left home	21 ○	Lost job or retired
15 ○	You left home	22 ○	Close relationship ended
16 ○	Close friend died	23 ○	Had major health problem.

Specify ONGOING SITUATIONS that you OFTEN FACE.

30 ○	Marital problems	35 ○	Pressure at work or school
31 ○	Financial problems	36 ○	Meeting family demands
32 ○	Sexual problems	37 ○	Coping with physical problems
33 ○	Trouble with relatives/friends	38 ○	Coping with emotional problems
34 ○	Trouble with co-workers	39 ○	Constantly facing deadlines

Specify REACTIONS that you EXPERIENCE FREQUENTLY.

(several times/week or more)

50 ○	Cold, sweaty palms	55 ○	Queasy stomach, "butterflies"
51 ○	Fast, pounding heart	56 ○	Feel highly irritable
52 ○	Tense shoulder, neck muscles	57 ○	Have trouble sleeping
53 ○	Clenching jaw	58 ○	Unable to relax
54 ○	Grinding teeth	59 ○	Unable to concentrate

Specify TRAITS which usually APPLY TO YOU.

60 ○	Never late	63 ○	Impatient
61 ○	Competitive	64 ○	Hard driving
62 ○	Rushed	65 ○	Rapid speech

HEALTH NEEDS and NOTIONS

Notion or statement	Strongly Agree 1 2 3 4 5 6 7 Strongly Disagree
70 Many illnesses can be prevented	①②③④⑤⑥⑦
71 People are responsible for their own health	①②③④⑤⑥⑦
72 If you feel good, you probably have no disease	①②③④⑤⑥⑦
73 Habits like smoking influence how long you live	①②③④⑤⑥⑦
74 Poor health largely results from bad luck	①②③④⑤⑥⑦
75 Doctors can do more about my health than I can	①②③④⑤⑥⑦
76 I can reduce my health risks	①②③④⑤⑥⑦

To what extent would your

health improvement efforts be	None or very little Lots or very much
77 Supported by your family	①②③④⑤⑥⑦
78 Supported by your friends	①②③④⑤⑥⑦
79 Supported by your community	①②③④⑤⑥⑦
80 Supported by your place of work	①②③④⑤⑥⑦

Mark programs in which you are interested.

81 ○	Alcohol control	87 ○	General health education
82 ○	Blood pressure management	88 ○	Human sexuality
83 ○	Cardiac rehab. program	89 ○	Nutrition counseling
84 ○	Diabetes management	90 ○	Smoking cessation
85 ○	Emotional problem counseling	91 ○	Stress management
86 ○	Exercise or fitness program	92 ○	Weight reduction

INFORMATION

Mark items for which you would like educational information.

10 ○ Alcohol		18 ○ Legal problems	
11 ○ Birth control		19 ○ Loneliness	
12 ○ Diet		20 ○ Marital problems	
13 ○ Drug abuse		21 ○ Medical emergencies	
14 ○ Emotional problems		22 ○ Self-breast exam	
15 ○ Exercise		23 ○ Sexual problems	
16 ○ Financial problems		24 ○ Smoking	
17 ○ Health hazards		25 ○ Venereal disease	

SELF-CARE

The early evaluation of symptoms, self-exams, and various professional health exams are important in detecting diseases. Regular medical follow-up is important in keeping problems under control and avoiding complications.

Yes No Have you-

30 ○ ○ Ever had a chest x-ray?
31 ○ ○ Had an abnormal chest x-ray?
32 ○ ○ Ever had an EKG (Electrocardiogram)?
33 ○ ○ Had an abnormal EKG?
34 ○ ○ Had a TB skin test?
35 ○ ○ Had a positive TB skin test?
36 ○ ○ Had eyes checked in past two years?
37 ○ ○ Had hearing tested (audiometry) in past two years?
38 ○ ○ Had dental exam in the past year?

Do you-

39 ○ ○ Regularly follow your physician's advice?
40 ○ ○ Plan annual medical symptom review with your physician or health service?
41 ○ ○ Plan annual rectal exam after age 30?

WOMEN *(Men go to "Tests")*

Yes No Do you or have you-

45 ○ ○ Had a PAP test within past year?
46 ○ ○ Had at least three PAP tests in past 5 years?
47 ○ ○ Had an abnormal PAP test in past?
48 ○ ○ Plan annual PAP tests in the future?
49 ○ ○ Check your breasts once a month for lumps?
50 ○ ○ Have a breast exam by a doctor once yearly?

TESTS

For these tests, if ever done, find out results from your physician. Mark values shown that are closest to your own results. If measured more than once, use most recent value.

Blood Pressure			Cholesterol
Systolic		Diastolic	
60 ○ 120 or less		65 ○ 82 or less	70 ○ 180 or less
61 ○ 140		66 ○ 88	71 ○ 210
62 ○ 160		67 ○ 94	72 ○ 240
63 ○ 180		68 ○ 100	73 ○ 270
64 ○ 200 or more		69 ○ 106 or more	74 ○ 300 or more

CONCLUSION

Yes No

80 ○ ○ Do you have any other problem not covered by this questionnaire?

Please give us your opinion of this system.

81 ○ Great   83 ○ Generally good, criticism minor
82 ○ Good   84 ○ Don't like it

Thanks for completing this questionnaire. Please review for accuracy, then mail or turn in according to instructions.

FOR OFFICE USE ONLY—To be completed by medical perse
Follow instructions printed on front cover of this questionnair

A. PHYSICAL MEASUREMENTS

10 Pulse Resting	11 Pulse Post Exercise	12 BP Resting	13 Ht. ft. in.

B. IMMUNIZATIONS
Enter year of last immunization. Leave not given or if uncertain.

20 DPT or Diph.	21 Tetanus Toxoid	22 Polio Oral	23 Mumps	24 Measles

Rubella titer Check instructions to see if this is required by facility. If required, the test must have been done within the

Results 30 ○ Positive (1:8 or greater)
31 ○ Negative (less than 1:8)

C. LABORATORY

Cholesterol		Triglycerides	Sug
40 Total	41 HDL	42	43 FBS

D. PHYSICAL EXAM

Yes No

50 ○ ○ Was physical exam done? If "Yes," go to 51.
51 ○ ○ Were there any abnormalities on physical exam?

4   © Medical Da

Health 80s Questionnaire

For Office Use Only			

3257023

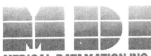

INSTRUCTIONS

Welcome to the world of HEALTH 80s! Completing this questionnaire will take only about half an hour of your time, and you will be getting back information designed to help you feel better and live longer. Please read the following instructions, then go ahead and fill out the questionnaire.

1. Use a black lead pencil.

2. Fill in the answer ovals completely. Keep all marks within the ovals. Do **NOT** make stray marks on the page.

3. Don't use checkmarks or "X's".

4. Many questions require a "yes" or "no" answer. Please mark one or the other.

5. Be as complete and accurate as you can. You may skip a question if you consider it too personal. However, remember that all information will be treated confidentially.

6. Cleanly erase any answer you want to change.

7. Don't fold, tear, or staple this form.

START with the IDENTIFICATION section below.

IDENTIFICATION Please print.

10 Today's Date ⬚⬚ - ⬚⬚ - ⬚⬚
Mo. Da. Yr.

11 Name ⬚⬚⬚⬚⬚⬚⬚⬚⬚⬚⬚⬚⬚⬚⬚⬚⬚⬚⬚⬚⬚⬚
Last Name, First Name, Middle Name

12 Social Security Number ⬚⬚⬚ - ⬚⬚ - ⬚⬚⬚⬚   13 ○ None

14 Birth Date ⬚⬚ - ⬚⬚ - ⬚⬚
Mo. Da. Yr.

15 ○ Female   16 ○ Male

17 Height ____ ft. ____ in.   18 Weight _____ lbs.

PERMANENT HOME ADDRESS

19 Street ⬚⬚⬚⬚⬚⬚⬚⬚⬚⬚⬚⬚⬚⬚⬚⬚⬚⬚⬚⬚⬚⬚⬚⬚

20 City ⬚⬚⬚⬚⬚⬚⬚⬚⬚⬚⬚⬚⬚⬚⬚⬚⬚⬚⬚⬚⬚⬚⬚

21 State or Province ⬚⬚⬚⬚⬚⬚⬚⬚⬚⬚⬚⬚⬚⬚⬚⬚⬚⬚⬚⬚

22 Zip ⬚⬚⬚⬚⬚

23 Country ⬚⬚⬚⬚⬚⬚⬚⬚⬚⬚⬚⬚⬚⬚⬚⬚⬚⬚⬚⬚⬚⬚

24 Telephone (Include area code) ⬚⬚⬚ - ⬚⬚⬚ - ⬚⬚⬚⬚   25 ○ None

DEMOGRAPHIC BACKG▮

Race
10 ○ American Indian
11 ○ Black
12 ○ Caucasian
13 ○ Other

Family Income Level
14 ○ Low
15 ○ Middle
16 ○ High

Marital Status
17 ○ Single
18 ○ Married
19 ○ Widowed
20 ○ Separated
21 ○ Divorced

ILLNESSES and MEDICAL PROBLEMS —

Yes No
○ ○ Have you had any of the problems listed below?

"Yes," mark items that apply. If "No," go to Disability section.

○ Alcoholism		40 ○ Fibrocystic breasts
○ Anemia		41 ○ Gallbladder prob.
○ Arthritis		42 ○ Hearing loss
○ Asthma		43 ○ High cholesterol
○ Back problem		44 ○ Hiatal hernia
○ Bronchitis, chronic		45 ○ High blood pressure
Cancer (mark type)		46 ○ High blood pressure,
○ Breast		uncontrolled
○ Cervix		47 ○ Hypoglycemia
○ Colon		48 ○ Kidney prob.
○ Leukemia		49 ○ Knee injury
○ Lung		50 ○ Mental illness
○ Prostate		51 ○ Migraine headache
○ Other cancer		52 ○ Obesity (more than
Cardiac or heart prob.		20 lbs. overweight)
○ Coronary disease		53 ○ Ovarian cyst
○ Enlarged heart		54 ○ Pelvic infection
○ Heart attack		55 ○ Peptic ulcer
○ Heart failure		56 ○ Phlebitis
○ Heart rhythm prob.		57 ○ Pneumonia
○ Rheumatic heart		58 ○ Polyps in colon
○ Other heart prob.		59 ○ Prostate prob.
○ Cirrhosis		60 ○ Serious injury with
○ Cystitis, bladder infection		permanent damage
○ Colitis		61 ○ Stroke
○ Depression		62 ○ Suicide attempt
○ Diabetes		63 ○ Thyroid problem
○ Diabetes, uncontrolled		64 ○ Tension headaches
○ Emphysema		65 ○ Venereal disease
○ Epilepsy		66 ○ Other problem, not listed
○ Eye prob., uncorrectable		

Yes No DISABILITY and HEALTH STATUS, do you or have you
○ ○ Been refused insurance due to health problems?
○ ○ Have a permanent restriction in physical activity?
○ ○ Require use of a wheelchair?
○ ○ Have a loss of function of one eye, kidney, or testicle?
"Yes," specify. 74 ○ Eye 75 ○ Kidney 76 ○ Testicle

Yes No
○ ○ Do you have a PERMANENT MEDICAL DISABILITY?
"Yes," specify cause.

○ Blindness		86 ○ High blood pressure
○ Cancer		87 ○ Low back problem
○ Cerebral palsy		88 ○ Mental health problem
○ Chronic lung disease		89 ○ Multiple sclerosis
○ Diabetes		90 ○ Residuals of an injury
○ Deafness		91 ○ Stroke
○ Heart disease		92 ○ Other cause not listed

Yes No
○ ○ Have you been admitted to a HOSPITAL?
"Yes," specify reason(s).
○ Illness   97 ○ Operation
○ Injury   98 ○ Pregnancy
○ Mental illness 99 ○ Check up

Yes No
10 ○ ○ Do you have any ALLERGIES?
If "Yes," specify.

11 ○ Aspirin		16 ○ Pollens, ragweed
12 ○ Bee stings		17 ○ Sulfa
13 ○ Eggs		18 ○ Tetanus toxoid
14 ○ Molds, fungi		19 ○ Drug not listed
15 ○ Penicillin		20 ○ Other not listed

Yes No
21 ○ ○ Do you take any MEDICINES frequently or regularly?
If "Yes," mark medicines that apply.

22 ○ Antibiotic		31 ○ Estrogen, hormone
23 ○ Antihistamine		32 ○ Heart med.
24 ○ Arthritis med.		33 ○ High blood press. med.
25 ○ Asthma med.		34 ○ Insulin
26 ○ Blood thinner		35 ○ Nerve med.
27 ○ Birth control pill		36 ○ Pain med.
28 ○ Cortisone, steroid		37 ○ Sleeping pill
29 ○ Diabetic pill		38 ○ Thyroid med.
30 ○ Diuretic (water pill)		39 ○ Other not listed

Yes No
40 ○ ○ Have you had any OPERATIONS?
If "Yes," mark operations you've had.

41 ○ Appendix		49 ○ Hernia
42 ○ Back		50 ○ Hysterectomy
43 ○ Breast		51 ○ Kidney
44 ○ Colon		52 ○ Tonsillectomy
45 ○ C-section		53 ○ Tubal ligation
46 ○ D and C		54 ○ Vasectomy
47 ○ Gallbladder		55 ○ Operation for cancer
48 ○ Heart		56 ○ Other not listed

Yes No
60 ○ ○ Have you had any FRACTURES (broken bones)?
If "Yes," indicate bone(s) involved.

61 ○ Skull	67 ○ Collarbone	73 ○ Thigh
62 ○ Nose	68 ○ Arm	74 ○ Kneecap
63 ○ Jaw	69 ○ Forearm	75 ○ Leg
64 ○ Neck	70 ○ Wrist	76 ○ Ankle
65 ○ Back	71 ○ Hand	77 ○ Foot
66 ○ Pelvis	72 ○ Hip	78 ○ Other not listed

Yes No IMMUNIZATIONS and INFECTIONS, have you had -
80 ○ ○ German measles (rubella) or immunization for it?
81 ○ ○ Measles (rubeola) or immunization for it?
82 ○ ○ Mumps or immunization for it?
83 ○ ○ Polio oral immunization?
84 ○ ○ Tetanus toxoid immunization within past 10 years?

Yes No
85 ○ ○ Are you generally aware of your family medical history?
If "Yes," mark items that apply to your blood relatives.

86 ○ Alcoholism		92 ○ High blood pressure
87 ○ Anemia (sickle cell)		93 ○ Mental illness
88 ○ Bleeding trait		94 ○ Stroke
89 ○ Cancer		95 ○ Suicide
90 ○ Diabetes		96 ○ Tuberculosis
91 ○ Heart disease		

Mark items that apply to you.
97 ○ Father died of heart attack before age 60.
98 ○ Mother died of heart attack before age 60.
99 ○ Mother or sister had cancer of the breast.

REVIEW OF SYSTEMS

These items concern either existing conditions or symptoms that occurred within the past year.

Yes No In the past year, have you had-

Head, Neurologic

10 ○ ○ Staggering or balance problems?
11 ○ ○ Spinning sensation or dizziness?
12 ○ ○ Fainting spells?
13 ○ ○ Convulsions or seizures?
14 ○ ○ Muscular twitching?
15 ○ ○ Memory problems?
16 ○ ○ Numbness or tingling in arm(s)?
17 ○ ○ Numbness or tingling in leg(s)?
18 ○ ○ Frequent or severe headaches?

Eyes

20 ○ ○ Persistent pain right eye?
21 ○ ○ Persistent pain left eye?
22 ○ ○ Persistent watering or itching of eyes?
23 ○ ○ Red, sore eyelids?
24 ○ ○ Double vision?
25 ○ ○ Unexplained decrease in vision in one eye?

Ears, Nose & Throat

30 ○ ○ Frequent earaches?
31 ○ ○ Sore or itching ear canals?
32 ○ ○ Frequent stuffy or runny nose?
33 ○ ○ Frequent postnasal drip, tickle in throat?
34 ○ ○ Persistent or frequent hoarseness?
35 ○ ○ Persistent sore tongue?
36 ○ ○ Bleeding or sore gums?
37 ○ ○ Tender swelling at base of teeth (abscess)?
38 ○ ○ Frequent toothaches or bad teeth?

Respiratory

40 ○ ○ Frequent or persistent wheezing?
41 ○ ○ Frequent or persistent cough?
42 ○ ○ Frequent or severe shortness of breath?
43 ○ ○ Shortness of breath that interferes with work or routine activities?

Cardiovascular

50 ○ ○ Shortness of breath lying down, relieved by sitting up?
51 ○ ○ Fluid retention with swelling of feet or legs?
52 ○ ○ Episodic pain, whiteness of hands or feet?
53 ○ ○ Calf pain when walking, relieved by rest?
54 ○ ○ Irregular heartbeat, skipped beats?
55 ○ ○ Bouts of heartbeat so fast you can't count?
56 ○ ○ Pain, pressure, or tight feeling in chest which forced you to stop walking?
57 ○ ○ Frequent or severe chest pain?

Digestive

60 ○ ○ Frequent nausea or vomiting?
61 ○ ○ Vomiting of blood?
62 ○ ○ Trouble swallowing solids?
63 ○ ○ Hot burning fluid in throat or chest?
64 ○ ○ Black tarry stools?
65 ○ ○ Frequent diarrhea or watery stools?
66 ○ ○ Frequent constipation?
67 ○ ○ Unexplained rectal bleeding?
68 ○ ○ Frequent or severe heartburn or indigestion?
69 ○ ○ Frequent or severe abdominal pain?

In the past year, have you had-

Yes No **Urinary**

10 ○ ○ Loss of urine control?
11 ○ ○ Awaken from sleep to urinate frequently?
12 ○ ○ Urinate more than 10 times a day?
13 ○ ○ Frequent urinary burning sensation?
14 ○ ○ Blood in urine?
15 ○ ○ Pain in flank accompanied by fever?
16 ○ ○ Trouble getting urine started?

Men (Women go to 25)

20 ○ ○ Pus or drainage from penis?
21 ○ ○ Rupture or swelling in groin?
22 ○ ○ Nodule in testicle growing larger?

Women (Men go to 40)

25 ○ ○ Have you ever had a period?
26 ○ ○ Have you ever been pregnant?

Yes No In the past year, have you had-

31 ○ ○ Hard lump in breast?
32 ○ ○ Persistent vaginal itching or discharge?
33 ○ ○ Irregular periods?
34 ○ ○ Excessive bleeding with periods?
35 ○ ○ Bleeding or spotting between periods?
36 ○ ○ Vaginal bleeding after menopause (change of life)?

Musculoskeletal

40 ○ ○ Frequent or severe neck pain?
41 ○ ○ Frequent or severe back pain?
42 ○ ○ Pain or stiffness in joint due to injury?
43 ○ ○ Persistent joint pain not due to injury?

Other Systems

50 ○ ○ Frequent or constant thirst?
51 ○ ○ Weight loss not explained by diet?
52 ○ ○ Constant fatigue?
53 ○ ○ Skin lesion that won't heal?
54 ○ ○ Persistent rash or pimples?
55 ○ ○ Frequent hot flashes?
56 ○ ○ Unexplained fever or chills?

FEELINGS

Mark the frequency with which you have the feelings or problems listed by filling the oval in the appropriate column.

M-Most of time S-Some of time R-Rarely or none

	M	S	R	
60	○	○	◓	Feel sad, depressed?
61	○	○	◓	Feel lonely?
62	○	○	◓	Wish to end it all?
63	○	○	◓	Still tired after a night's sleep?
64	○	○	◓	Feel tense and anxious?
65	○	○	◓	Worry about things generally?
66	○	○	◓	More aggressive, hard-driving than friends?
67	○	○	◓	Have an intense desire to achieve?
68	○	○	◓	Greatly upset by criticism?
69	○	○	◓	Feel optimistic about the future?
70	○	○	◓	Have feelings of inadequacy?
71	○	○	◓	Feel someone is out to get you?

4

5-215

LITY OF LIFE

quality is a complex issue related to both physical and emotional well-being. Among other things, it hinges on your comfort or satisfaction with self, your relations with others, your ability to meet the demands of life, and your ability to enjoy things. This section covers some of these life quality -minants. For each topic indicate your usual current status, what you feel you could realistically attain (optimal level), and the importance you attach to opic. Note that the numeric "Degree Scale" allows you to grade your responses from "1" (Low or Poor) to "7" (High or Good).

MFORT WITH YOURSELF

	Low or Poor	High or Good
sfaction with physical appearance		
Your current level	①②③④⑤⑥⑦	
Level possible for you to attain	①②③④⑤⑥⑦	
Importance to you	①②③④⑤⑥⑦	
r physical health generally		
Your current level	①②③④⑤⑥⑦	
Level possible for you to attain	①②③④⑤⑥⑦	
Importance to you	①②③④⑤⑥⑦	
dency to practice healthy habits		
Your current level	①②③④⑤⑥⑦	
Level possible for you to attain	①②③④⑤⑥⑦	
Importance to you	①②③④⑤⑥⑦	
r emotional well-being		
Your current level	①②③④⑤⑥⑦	
Level possible for you to attain	①②③④⑤⑥⑦	
Importance to you	①②③④⑤⑥⑦	
-confidence		
Your current level	①②③④⑤⑥⑦	
Level possible for you to attain	①②③④⑤⑥⑦	
Importance to you	①②③④⑤⑥⑦	
-respect, self-image		
Your current level	①②③④⑤⑥⑦	
Level possible for you to attain	①②③④⑤⑥⑦	
Importance to you	①②③④⑤⑥⑦	

MFORT WITH OTHERS

	Low or Poor	High or Good
lity to express yourself, make needs known		
Your current level	①②③④⑤⑥⑦	
Level possible for you to attain	①②③④⑤⑥⑦	
Importance to you	①②③④⑤⑥⑦	
lity to listen to others, understand		
Your current level	①②③④⑤⑥⑦	
Level possible for you to attain	①②③④⑤⑥⑦	
Importance to you	①②③④⑤⑥⑦	
lity to give and receive love		
Your current level	①②③④⑤⑥⑦	
Level possible for you to attain	①②③④⑤⑥⑦	
Importance to you	①②③④⑤⑥⑦	
lity to get along with others		
Your current level	①②③④⑤⑥⑦	
Level possible for you to attain	①②③④⑤⑥⑦	
Importance to you	①②③④⑤⑥⑦	
lity to maintain lasting relationships		
Your current level	①②③④⑤⑥⑦	
Level possible for you to attain	①②③④⑤⑥⑦	
Importance to you	①②③④⑤⑥⑦	
nse of belonging, of having "roots"		
Your current level	①②③④⑤⑥⑦	
Level possible for you to attain	①②③④⑤⑥⑦	
Importance to you	①②③④⑤⑥⑦	

MEETING THE DEMANDS OF LIFE

		Low or Poor	High or Good
	Ability to accept responsibility		
10	Your current level	①②③④⑤⑥⑦	
11	Level possible for you to attain	①②③④⑤⑥⑦	
12	Importance to you	①②③④⑤⑥⑦	
	Ability to solve problems, make decisions		
13	Your current level	①②③④⑤⑥⑦	
14	Level possible for you to attain	①②③④⑤⑥⑦	
15	Importance to you	①②③④⑤⑥⑦	
	Tendency to follow through, get jobs done		
16	Your current level	①②③④⑤⑥⑦	
17	Level possible for you to attain	①②③④⑤⑥⑦	
18	Importance to you	①②③④⑤⑥⑦	
	Ability to adapt, be flexible		
19	Your current level	①②③④⑤⑥⑦	
20	Level possible for you to attain	①②③④⑤⑥⑦	
21	Importance to you	①②③④⑤⑥⑦	
	Ability to cope with health risks, problems		
22	Your current level	①②③④⑤⑥⑦	
23	Level possible for you to attain	①②③④⑤⑥⑦	
24	Importance to you	①②③④⑤⑥⑦	
	Ability to cope with problems of living		
25	Your current level	①②③④⑤⑥⑦	
26	Level possible for you to attain	①②③④⑤⑥⑦	
27	Importance to you	①②③④⑤⑥⑦	

ENJOYMENT OF LIFE

		Low or Poor	High or Good
	Time available for recreation, leisure		
30	Your current level	①②③④⑤⑥⑦	
31	Level possible for you to attain	①②③④⑤⑥⑦	
32	Importance to you	①②③④⑤⑥⑦	
	Enjoyment of recreational activities		
33	Your current level	①②③④⑤⑥⑦	
34	Level possible for you to attain	①②③④⑤⑥⑦	
35	Importance to you	①②③④⑤⑥⑦	
	Enjoyment of work or school		
36	Your current level	①②③④⑤⑥⑦	
37	Level possible for you to attain	①②③④⑤⑥⑦	
38	Importance to you	①②③④⑤⑥⑦	
	Enjoyment of relationships with family, friends		
39	Your current level	①②③④⑤⑥⑦	
40	Level possible for you to attain	①②③④⑤⑥⑦	
41	Importance to you	①②③④⑤⑥⑦	
	Enjoyment of community, environment		
42	Your current level	①②③④⑤⑥⑦	
43	Level possible for you to attain	①②③④⑤⑥⑦	
44	Importance to you	①②③④⑤⑥⑦	
	Level of spiritual fulfillment		
45	Your current level	①②③④⑤⑥⑦	
46	Level possible for you to attain	①②③④⑤⑥⑦	
47	Importance to you	①②③④⑤⑥⑦	

HABITS and RISK FACTORS

Your habits influence your ability to achieve and maintain good health and long life.

EATING

Yes	No	Do you usually or generally-
10 ○	○	Consider yourself overweight?
11 ○	○	Follow a restricted diet for medical reasons?
12 ○	○	Eat 3 meals a day?
13 ○	○	Snack between meals?
14 ○	○	Know what foods are high in carbohydrates, starches?
15 ○	○	Know what foods are high in cholesterol?
16 ○	○	Know what foods are high in fiber?
17 ○	○	Know the difference between saturated and unsaturated fats?
18 ○	○	Know how to count calories accurately without the aid of a book?
19 ○	○	Eat fried foods 5 or more times per week?
20 ○	○	Eat "out" 5 or more times per week (food not cooked at home)?

Specify number of servings you eat during a typical DAY (24 hrs.)

DAILY BASIS-

Type of food	DON'T EAT	Usual servings per DAY- 1 or less 2 3 4 5 6more 7 or
31 Fruit or fruit juice	○	① ② ③ ④ ⑤ ⑥ ⑦
32 Vegetables	○	① ② ③ ④ ⑤ ⑥ ⑦
33 Cereal-non pre-sweetened	○	① ② ③ ④ ⑤ ⑥ ⑦
34 Bread, rolls, biscuits, bagels	○	① ② ③ ④ ⑤ ⑥ ⑦
35 White bread, rolls, biscuits	○	① ② ③ ④ ⑤ ⑥ ⑦
36 Potatoes, rice, macaroni, pastas	○	① ② ③ ④ ⑤ ⑥ ⑦
37 Pie, cake, doughnuts, sweet rolls	○	① ② ③ ④ ⑤ ⑥ ⑦
38 Meat or meat substitutes-beef, pork, cheese, poultry, fish	○	① ② ③ ④ ⑤ ⑥ ⑦
39 Soybeans, lentils, legumes, nuts, peanut butter	○	① ② ③ ④ ⑤ ⑥ ⑦
40 Skim milk	○	① ② ③ ④ ⑤ ⑥ ⑦
41 2% milk	○	① ② ③ ④ ⑤ ⑥ ⑦
42 Whole milk	○	① ② ③ ④ ⑤ ⑥ ⑦
43 Butter, margarine (tsp.)	○	① ② ③ ④ ⑤ ⑥ ⑦
44 Soft drinks (regular, non-diet)	○	① ② ③ ④ ⑤ ⑥ ⑦
45 Caffeinated coffee, tea, cola	○	① ② ③ ④ ⑤ ⑥ ⑦
46 Beer or wine	○	① ② ③ ④ ⑤ ⑥ ⑦
47 Salt (shaker use)	○	① ② ③ ④ ⑤ ⑥ ⑦
48 Pretzels, crackers	○	① ② ③ ④ ⑤ ⑥ ⑦
49 Potato or corn chips, french fries	○	① ② ③ ④ ⑤ ⑥ ⑦
50 Sugar (tsp.)	○	① ② ③ ④ ⑤ ⑥ ⑦

Specify number of servings you eat during a typical WEEK (7 days).
Keep in mind there are 21 meals/week.

WEEKLY BASIS

Type of Food	DON'T EAT	Usual servings per WEEK- 1 or less 2 3 4 5 6more 7 or
51 Beef or lamb	○	① ② ③ ④ ⑤ ⑥ ⑦
52 Pork, bacon, sausage	○	① ② ③ ④ ⑤ ⑥ ⑦
53 Weiners, lunchmeats	○	① ② ③ ④ ⑤ ⑥ ⑦
54 Poultry or fish	○	① ② ③ ④ ⑤ ⑥ ⑦
55 Shrimp, lobster, clams	○	① ② ③ ④ ⑤ ⑥ ⑦
56 Eggs	○	① ② ③ ④ ⑤ ⑥ ⑦
57 Hard cheese	○	① ② ③ ④ ⑤ ⑥ ⑦
58 Cottage cheese, soft cheese	○	① ② ③ ④ ⑤ ⑥ ⑦
59 Ice Cream, milk shakes	○	① ② ③ ④ ⑤ ⑥ ⑦
60 Salad oil, sour cream, mayonnaise	○	① ② ③ ④ ⑤ ⑥ ⑦
61 Candy	○	① ② ③ ④ ⑤ ⑥ ⑦

EXERCISE

Yes	No	Do you-
10 ○	○	Know the type of exercise that may help to prevent heart attacks?
11 ○	○	Know how to take your own pulse and monitor the effects of exercise?
12 ○	○	Get regular strenuous exercise, such as jogging, for at least 20 minutes 3 times a week?
13 ○	○	Get regular exercise of any type?

If "Yes" to item 13, complete the section below. If "No," go to item 40

	Don't Do This	Frequency (DAYS per WEEK) 1 2 3 4 5 6 7	Length ses (MINU DA 10 20
14 Walking slow (20 min/mile)	○	① ② ③ ④ ⑤ ⑥ ⑦	⑩ ⑳ ⓪
15 Walking fast (15 min/mile)	○	① ② ③ ④ ⑤ ⑥ ⑦	⑩ ⑳ ⓪
16 Jogging (10 min/mile)	○	① ② ③ ④ ⑤ ⑥ ⑦	⑩ ⑳ ⓪
17 Running (8 min/mile)	○	① ② ③ ④ ⑤ ⑥ ⑦	⑩ ⑳ ⓪
18 Cycling slow (6 mph)	○	① ② ③ ④ ⑤ ⑥ ⑦	⑩ ⑳ ⓪
19 Cycling fast (12 mph)	○	① ② ③ ④ ⑤ ⑥ ⑦	⑩ ⑳ ⓪
20 Swimming slow (25 yds/min)	○	① ② ③ ④ ⑤ ⑥ ⑦	⑩ ⑳ ⓪
21 Swimming fast (50 yds/min)	○	① ② ③ ④ ⑤ ⑥ ⑦	⑩ ⑳ ⓪
Racquet sports			
22 Recreational or doubles	○	① ② ③ ④ ⑤ ⑥ ⑦	⑩ ⑳ ⓪
23 Competitive or singles	○	① ② ③ ④ ⑤ ⑥ ⑦	⑩ ⑳ ⓪
24 Calisthenics	○	① ② ③ ④ ⑤ ⑥ ⑦	⑩ ⑳ ⓪
25 Dancing	○	① ② ③ ④ ⑤ ⑥ ⑦	⑩ ⑳ ⓪
26 Basketball, football, soccer or similar sport	○	① ② ③ ④ ⑤ ⑥ ⑦	⑩ ⑳ ⓪
27 Weight training	○	① ② ③ ④ ⑤ ⑥ ⑦	⑩ ⑳ ⓪
28 Golf or bowling	○	① ② ③ ④ ⑤ ⑥ ⑦	⑩ ⑳ ⓪
29 Downhill skiing in season	○	① ② ③ ④ ⑤ ⑥ ⑦	⑩ ⑳ ⓪
30 Cross country skiing in season	○	① ② ③ ④ ⑤ ⑥ ⑦	⑩ ⑳ ⓪

SMOKING

Yes	No	Do you-
40 ○	○	Smoke a pipe and inhale 5 or more times/day?
41 ○	○	Smoke cigars and inhale 5 or more times/day?
42 ○	○	Have you ever smoked cigarettes?

If yes, specify amount and duration.

Daily amount	Number of years
43 ○ 1/2 pack/day or less	47 ○ Less than 1 year
44 ○ 1/2 to 1 pack/day	48 ○ 1 to 5 years
45 ○ 1 to 2 packs/day	49 ○ 5 to 10 years
46 ○ Over 2 packs/day	50 ○ Over 10 years

Yes	No	
51 ○	○	Do you currently smoke cigarettes?

If you used to smoke cigarettes, but stopped, specify number of years since you stopped.

52 ○ 1 yr.	55 ○ 4 yrs.	58 ○ 7 yrs.
53 ○ 2 yrs.	56 ○ 5 yrs.	59 ○ 8 yrs.
54 ○ 3 yrs.	57 ○ 6 yrs.	60 ○ 9 or more

COHOL

Yes No
○   ○ Do you currently drink alcohol?
○   ○ Did you formerly drink alcohol but stopped?

ou have ever drunk alcohol, specify details.

icate the number of drinks consumed during a typical drinking
asion (a drink is a bottle of beer, a shot of whiskey, or equivalent).

○ 1 to 2 drinks   14 ○ 6 to 10 drinks
○ 2 to 6 drinks   15 ○ Over 10 drinks

the average, indicate the amount and duration at this level.

Amount per week		Number of years
○ Less than 2 drinks/wk.	21 ○	Less than one year
○ 2 to 10 drinks/wk.	22 ○	1 to 5 years
○ 10 to 25 drinks/wk.	23 ○	5 to 10 years
○ 25 to 40 drinks/wk.	24 ○	10 to 20 years
○ Over 40 drinks/wk.	25 ○	Over 20 years

UGS

Yes No Do you-
○   ○ Know the short and long term effects of street drugs?
○   ○ Have a problem with drugs?
○   ○ Want help with drug counseling?

AUMA, ACCIDENTS and OTHER HAZARDS

Yes No Do you, or are you-
○   ○ Frequently exposed to industrial chemicals?
○   ○ Frequently exposed to insecticides and pesticides?
○   ○ Exposed to loud noise without ear protection?
○   ○ Operate or work around industrial or farm machinery?
○   ○ Climb or work on ladders, scaffolds?
○   ○ Water ski or boat without a life preserver?
○   ○ Know how to swim?
○   ○ Live in an area where violent crime is common?
○   ○ Know how to give basic first aid, life support (CPR,
            cardiac resuscitation, mouth-to-mouth breathing)?
○   ○ Drive after drinking alcohol or taking drugs?
○   ○ Ride with drivers who have been drinking alcohol
            or taking drugs?
○   ○ Tend to exceed the speed limit?

ow many miles do you travel in a car or other motor vehicle each
ear (average is 12,000 miles)?

○ Up to 10,000   44 ○ 15,000 to 20,000
○ 10,000 to 15,000   45 ○ Over 20,000

hat percent of the time do you wear a seat belt?

○ 0 to 25%   48 ○ 50% to 75%
○ 25% to 50%   49 ○ 75% to 100%

hat percent of the time do you wear a shoulder strap?

○ 0 to 25%   52 ○ 50 to 75%
○ 25% to 50%   53 ○ 75% to 100%

8-802

STRESS

Specify CHANGES that have occurred in your life in the PAST YEAR.

10 ○ Spouse died   17 ○ Got divorced or separated
11 ○ Close family member died   18 ○ Lost a lot of money
12 ○ Moved to a new town   19 ○ Took on a lot of debt
13 ○ Changed jobs   20 ○ Got married
14 ○ Son/daughter left home   21 ○ Lost job or retired
15 ○ You left home   22 ○ Close relationship ended
16 ○ Close friend died   23 ○ Had major health problem.

Specify ONGOING SITUATIONS that you OFTEN FACE.

30 ○ Marital problems   35 ○ Pressure at work or school
31 ○ Financial problems   36 ○ Meeting family demands
32 ○ Sexual problems   37 ○ Coping with physical problems
33 ○ Trouble with relatives/friends 38 ○ Coping with emotional problems
34 ○ Trouble with co-workers   39 ○ Constantly facing deadlines

Specify REACTIONS that you EXPERIENCE FREQUENTLY.
(several times/week or more)

50 ○ Cold, sweaty palms   55 ○ Queasy stomach, "butterflies"
51 ○ Fast, pounding heart   56 ○ Feel highly irritable
52 ○ Tense shoulder, neck muscles 57 ○ Have trouble sleeping
53 ○ Clenching jaw   58 ○ Unable to relax
54 ○ Grinding teeth   59 ○ Unable to concentrate

Specify TRAITS which usually APPLY TO YOU.

60 ○ Never late   63 ○ Impatient
61 ○ Competitive   64 ○ Hard driving
62 ○ Rushed   65 ○ Rapid speech

HEALTH NEEDS and NOTIONS

		Strongly Agree						Strongly Disagree
Notion or statement		1	2	3	4	5	6	7
70	Many illnesses can be prevented	①	②	③	④	⑤	⑥	⑦
71	People are responsible for their own health	①	②	③	④	⑤	⑥	⑦
72	If you feel good, you probably have no disease	①	②	③	④	⑤	⑥	⑦
73	Habits like smoking influence how long you live	①	②	③	④	⑤	⑥	⑦
74	Poor health largely results from bad luck	①	②	③	④	⑤	⑥	⑦
75	Doctors can do more about my health than I can	①	②	③	④	⑤	⑥	⑦
76	I can reduce my health risks	①	②	③	④	⑤	⑥	⑦

To what extent would your health improvement efforts be	None or very little					Lots or very much
77 Supported by your family	①	②	③	④	⑤	⑥
78 Supported by your friends	①	②	③	④	⑤	⑥
79 Supported by your community	①	②	③	④	⑤	⑥
80 Supported by your place of work	①	②	③	④	⑤	⑥

Mark programs in which you are interested.

81 ○ Alcohol control   87 ○ General health education
82 ○ Blood pressure management 88 ○ Human sexuality
83 ○ Cardiac rehab. program   89 ○ Nutrition counseling
84 ○ Diabetes management   90 ○ Smoking cessation
85 ○ Emotional problem counseling 91 ○ Stress management
86 ○ Exercise or fitness program 92 ○ Weight reduction

INFORMATION

Mark items for which you would like educational information.

10 ○ Alcohol			18 ○ Legal problems	
11 ○ Birth control			19 ○ Loneliness	
12 ○ Diet			20 ○ Marital problems	
13 ○ Drug abuse			21 ○ Medical emergencies	
14 ○ Emotional problems			22 ○ Self-breast exam	
15 ○ Exercise			23 ○ Sexual problems	
16 ○ Financial problems			24 ○ Smoking	
17 ○ Health hazards			25 ○ Venereal disease	

SELF-CARE

The early evaluation of symptoms, self-exams, and various professional health exams are important in detecting diseases. Regular medical follow-up is important in keeping problems under control and avoiding complications.

Yes No Have you—

30 ○	○	Ever had a chest x-ray?
31 ○	○	Had an abnormal chest x-ray?
32 ○	○	Ever had an EKG (Electrocardiogram)?
33 ○	○	Had an abnormal EKG?
34 ○	○	Had a TB skin test?
35 ○	○	Had a positive TB skin test?
36 ○	○	Had eyes checked in past two years?
37 ○	○	Had hearing tested (audiometry) in past two years?
38 ○	○	Had dental exam in the past year?

Do you—

39 ○	○	Regularly follow your physician's advice?
40 ○	○	Plan annual medical symptom review with your physician or health service?
41 ○	○	Plan annual rectal exam after age 30?

WOMEN *(Men go to "Tests")*

Yes No Do you or have you—

45 ○	○	Had a PAP test within past year?
46 ○	○	Had at least three PAP tests in past 5 years?
47 ○	○	Had an abnormal PAP test in past?
48 ○	○	Plan annual PAP tests in the future?
49 ○	○	Check your breasts once a month for lumps?
50 ○	○	Have a breast exam by a doctor once yearly?

TESTS

For these tests, if ever done, find out results from your physician. Mark values shown that are closest to your own results. If measured more than once, use most recent value.

Blood Pressure		Cholesterol
Systolic	Diastolic	
60 ○ 120 or less	65 ○ 82 or less	70 ○ 180 or less
61 ○ 140	66 ○ 88	71 ○ 210
62 ○ 160	67 ○ 94	72 ○ 240
63 ○ 180	68 ○ 100	73 ○ 270
64 ○ 200 or more	69 ○ 106 or more	74 ○ 300 or more

CONCLUSION

Yes No

80 ○ ○ Do you have any other problem not covered by this questionnaire?

Please give us your opinion of this system.

81 ○ Great	83 ○ Generally good, criticism minor
82 ○ Good	84 ○ Don't like it

Thanks for completing this questionnaire. **Please review for accuracy, then mail or turn in according to instructions.**

FOR OFFICE USE ONLY—To be completed by medical personnel only. Follow instructions printed on front cover of this questionnaire.

A. PHYSICAL MEASUREMENTS

10 Pulse Resting	11 Pulse Post Exercise	12 BP Resting	13 Ht. ft. in.	14 Wt. lbs.

B. IMMUNIZATIONS

Enter year of last immunization. Leave blank if not given or if uncertain.

20 DPT or Diph.	21 Tetanus Toxoid	22 Polio Oral	23 Mumps	24 Measles	25 Rubella

Rubella titer Check instructions to see if this is required by the facility. If required, the test must have been done within the past year.

Results 30 ○ Positive (1:8 or greater)
　　　　31 ○ Negative (less than 1:8)

C. LABORATORY

Cholesterol		Triglycerides	Sugar	
40 Total	41 HDL	42	43 FBS	44 2HrPC

D. PHYSICAL EXAM

Yes No

50 ○	○	Was physical exam done? If "Yes," go to 51.
51 ○	○	Were there any abnormalities on physical exam?

HEALTH HISTORY REPORT   MARKETING

ROBERTS, JASON   Date Completed: 05-02-81
Age 41   Male   Questionnaire: 1600   2753042
DOB: 06-01-40   Enter:
SS#: 621-54-1198   Class:
HT: 6' 1"   Occupation: ACCOUNTANT
WT: 220 lbs.
                                  Emergency Notification.
Home Address: ROBERTS, SARAH
876 FAIRWAY LANE   WIFE
SPRING VALLEY, ME 54221   Address not specified
Phone: 207-634-2279
                                  Phone: Not specified
Health Insurance:
METROPOLITAN   Family Physician:
Policy No: 7564127 A   PAULSON, B. DR.

DEMOGRAPHIC....... Born USA, USA citizen, Caucasian, married,
                   children (3), older siblings (1), younger
                   siblings (2), grew up in urban area, middle income
                   level, physical health good, emotional health good.
ILLNESSES......... Visual pb corrected with glasses or contacts,
                   cholecystitis.
MEDICATIONS....... Diuretic, other not listed.
HOSPITALIZATIONS... Check-up (1), in past year, check-up.   (?)
OPERATIONS........ Appendectomy, tonsillectomy
IMMUN/INFECT...... Immun: DPT, diphtheria, German measles, measles,
                   mumps, oral polio, smallpox, tetanus, received
                   tetanus immunization 6 or more yrs ago.
FAMILY HX .... Alcoholism, cancer, hypertension, hyperlipidemia.
DIGESTIVE......... Indigestion.
NUTRITION......... Average daily intake = 1840 calories. Eats fried
                   food 5x/week or more.
EXERCISE.......... Average daily expenditure - 30 calories. Does not
                   get regular strenuous exercise.
TRAUMA/HAZARDS..... Drives up to 10,000 miles/year, wears seatbelt
                   75-100% of time, wears shoulder strap 75-100% of
                   time.
STRESS............ Stress level = 47 (moderately high).
ATTITUDES......... Health misconception level = 14 (moderate).
                   Support level = 17 (good).
PROGRAMS.......... BP management, nutrition.
SELF-CARE......... Chest x-ray, EKG, TB skin test.
TESTS............. BP 120 or less/82 or less, cholesterol 210 mg%.
OPINION OF SYSTEM.. Great.
PULSE, BP......... BP : 160/90

NOTE: *** STRESS LEVEL - 47 (MODERATELY HIGH)

Sections coded (?) contain incomplete or uncertain responses.

ROBERTS, JASON   HEALTH HISTORY REPORT   6- 5-81

Your Health Risk Index

MEDICAL DATAMATION
SOUTHWEST AND HARRISON   BELLEVUE, OHIO 44811

ROBERTS, JASON E.
876 FAIRWAY LANE
SPRING VALLEY, ME 54221

Date: 12/11/79
Number: 800- 1234567
Birthdate: 2/ 1/40
Ht: 6' 1"   Wt: 205 lbs.
BP: 160/94 Chol: 240 mg%

Your HEALTH RISKS and CONTRIBUTING FACTORS

FOR THE NEXT 30 YEARS
Causes of Death and Contributing Factors

		RISK OF DYING		
		Yours	Average	Achievable
1	Coronary heart disease	24.4%	13.5%	5.6%
	Factors: Blood pressure, cholesterol, exercise habits, family history, weight			
2	Stroke	2.5	1.5	0.7
	Factors: Blood pressure, cholesterol			
3	Cirrhosis	1.6	1.6	0.3
	Factors: Alcohol habits			
4	Suicide	1.1	1.1	1.1
	Factors: None identified			
5	Motor vehicle accident	0.9	1.0	0.5
	Factors: Alcohol habits, mileage			
6	Cancer of colon	0.9	0.9	0.3
	Factors: No rectal exam			
7	Arterial disease	0.8	0.5	0.2
	Factors: Blood pressure, cholesterol			
8	Cancer of lungs	0.7	3.4	0.7
	Factors: None identified			
	Other causes	12.3	12.8	12.3
	TOTAL RISK OF DYING IN NEXT 30 YEARS	45.2%	36.3%	21.7%

Your LIFE EXPECTANCY PREDICTIONS

Comparative Ages		Life Expectations -	Life Remaining	Total Lifespan
Actual Age	39.8 yrs.	For an *average* person of your age, race, sex	33.5 yrs.	73.3 yrs.
Health Age	42.3 yrs.	For *you* based on your current analysis	31.3 yrs.	71.1 yrs.
Achievable Age	31.5 yrs.	For *you* based on maximum risk reduction	41.2 yrs.	81.0 yrs.
		Potential gain in *your* life expectancy	+ 9.9 yrs.	+ 9.9 yrs.

HOW *You* CAN LIVE LONGER

Rank	Actions You Can Take	Gain in Life Expectancy
1	Reduce, control cholesterol level	3.4 yrs.
2	Reduce, control high blood pressure	2.5 yrs.
3	Follow a program of regular vigorous exercise	1.4 yrs.
4	Reduce weight to 165, maintain	0.5 yrs.
5	Limit alcohol to 2 drinks/week	0.3 yrs.
6	Get annual rectal exam after age 30	0.2 yrs.
7	Reduce mileage to less than 10,000 miles/yr if possible	0.1 yrs.
8	Added benefit from doing ALL of the above	1.5 yrs.

TOTAL GAIN IN LIFE EXPECTANCY   + 9.9 yrs.

HEALTH RISK INDEX

Background

During the last 20 years, medical and actuarial experts developed a health education tool known as "health hazard appraisal" to help people identify and reduce their health risks. This technique forms the basis of your Health Risk Index. Causes of death by age, sex, and race are analyzed in terms of contributing causes. Group statistics are applied to individuals so that a person can identify his risk of dying by various causes, take note of contributing factors, and follow through on improving his chances of staying alive and healthy by taking risk reduction actions.

Your Health Risks and Contributing Factors

Health risks are problems or conditions that can kill you. This section lists possible causes of your death in order of decreasing frequency for the time period shown. Risk of dying during that period of time is expressed on a percentage basis. Your risk is based on your current analysis and is derived from information you supplied in your health questionnaire. The risk of an average person of your age, sex and race is shown for comparison. Your achievable risk indicates a favorable change in your chances of living based on risk reduction actions you can take.

Contributing factors to your possible causes of death stem from a variety of sources, including your habits, family medical history, and existing conditions such as high blood pressure. Some factors cannot be altered, such as having a family history of heart attack. However, many factors can be altered favorably and your risk of dying reduced by actions that you take.

Your risk of dying is determined for a specific period of time. This period of time is dependent on your age. Generally, young people are interested in both their chances of reaching middle age and in how long they will live. For young people, the Health Risk Index projects risks for two time periods, one for reaching middle age and one for a "lifetime." For people who are already nearing middle age or beyond, risks are projected for only one time period. In any case, the goal is to present you with information which will be useful to you in reducing your risks.

Your Life Expectancy Predictions

How old are you in terms of your health risks, and how long are you likely to live? This section answers these questions and suggests how much your "age" and life expectancy might be improved. Your actual age is your real or chronologic age. The years of life remaining and total lifespan for an average person of this age are shown. Your health age is based on your current risk level; it was determined through calculating your years of life remaining and total lifespan. For instance, if you are 25 years old and have a health age of 30, you might expect to live the same number of years as the average 30-year-old person (instead of the average 25-year-old). If you are 25 and have a health age of 20, you are better off than the average person your age and can expect to live as long as the average 20-year-old.

Your achievable age was determined by considering your life expectancy in terms of what it would be like should you now reduce all risks possible and continue to follow through on these risk reduction actions in the future. If you are 25 years old, have a health age of 30, and an achievable age of 20, it means you can have the life expectancy of an average 20-year-old rather than a 30-year-old. Your potential gain in life expectancy is shown on the bottom line of this section. NOTE: Your actual age should be added to your life remaining in any category to obtain your total lifespan in that category.

How To Live Longer

Specific actions for you to take to reduce your risks and improve your life expectancy are listed here. Actions are listed in order of decreasing importance with regard to impact on your life expectancy. Please note that the gain shown is entirely dependent on you and what actions you take now and continue to follow through on. These actions generally take one of three forms: 1) eliminating a dangerous habit, such as smoking; 2) starting a healthy habit, like getting regular exercise; or 3) keeping a condition under control, such as high blood pressure or obesity. Most of these actions will not only improve your life expectancy, but allow you to feel better during the rest of your life.

Conclusion

The Health Risk Index does not show all health hazards. It deals only with those that have been studied enough to use in making reasonable predictions regarding their effect on health. Many other hazards are known, but they have not been sufficiently studied to permit reasonable predictive analysis. There are many other hazards that are suspected, and probably many more that are yet unknown. However, health care professionals must use information and tools that are available now in an effort to prevent problems from arising, or keeping problems under control if they are already present. The Health Risk Index is an information tool that you can use to begin taking actions that will reduce your health risks. Health care professionals may assist you in understanding risk reduction techniques, but the motivation to take appropriate action rests with you.

Warranty

Medical Datamation warrants that this report is based on existing techniques for analyzing and applying national mortality statistics in conjunction with hazards contributing to the causes of death. It further warrants that such techniques are generally meaningful in regard to the health risks of individuals. However, Medical Datamation asserts that these techniques are subject to statistical variation, and that particular individuals may experience events differing from those specified in this report. Consequently, Medical Datamation makes no warranties regarding the application of this report to particular individuals or its use for specific purposes.

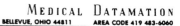

SOUTHWEST & HARRISON   BELLEVUE, OHIO 44811   AREA CODE 419 483-6060

EXERCISE

Regular, vigorous exercise reduces cardiovascular risks. To gain significant health benefits, exercise should occur at least four times per week and average 100 calories of energy expenditure or more per day (700 or more per week). Jogging 20 to 30 minutes every other day or walking 30 minutes or more daily would be sufficient to meet this goal.

YOUR RESULTS

Type	Min/day	Days/week	Cal/week	Av. Cal/day
Swimming, slow........20		1	170	20
TOTAL.....................................170				20

Please note: your weight, if available, has been considered in these calculations.

Your exercise level is very low. You are not obtaining much benefit to your health.

RECOMMENDATIONS

* INCREASE REGULAR VIGOROUS EXERCISE TO 100 CAL/DAY OR MORE.
* IF OUT OF SHAPE, START GRADUALLY AND BUILD UP TOLERANCE.
* CONSULT A PHYSICIAN BEFORE STARTING EXERCISE PROGRAM IF YOU HAVE A HEART CONDITION OR ANY OTHER SERIOUS HEALTH PROBLEM.

SMOKING

Congratulations on not smoking! You are avoiding substantial risks to your health. Keep it up!

TRAUMA/HAZARDS

You are doing a good job of reducing risks associated with trauma and other hazards!

STRESS

Events in people's lives produce stress, and stress can be harmful. The effects of stress depend upon the nature of the events and how well people cope with them. Chronic, intense stress can produce tension, anxiety, and physical symptoms and even contribute to serious problems such as coronary heart disease.

YOUR RESULTS

CHANGES
Child left home................3
Major health problem..........5
TOTAL (Moderate)..............8

SITUATIONS
Work, school pressure........6
Constant deadlines...........6
TOTAL (Moderately high)......12

TRAITS
Never late....................6
Rushed........................4
TOTAL (Moderate)..............10

REACTIONS
Fast, pounding heart.........7
Trouble sleeping............10
TOTAL (Moderately high)......17

OVERALL STRESS LEVEL: 47 (MODERATELY HIGH)

ROBERTS, JASON   LIFESTYLE INDEX   6/ 5/81

MEDICAL DATAMATION

SOUTHWEST & HARRISON   BELLEVUE, OHIO 44811   AREA CODE 419 483-6060

RECOMMENDATIONS
* ALTER ON-GOING SITUATIONS IF POSSIBLE TO REDUCE STRESS LEVEL.
* LEARN TO RECOGNIZE STRESS-RELATED SYMPTOMS AND REACTIONS.
* IMPROVE COPING SKILLS THROUGH STRESS MANAGEMENT TRAINING.

ATTITUDES & SUPPORT
    Many people mistakenly believe that they cannot influence their own
health. Actually, personal behavior or lifestyle is one of the primary
determinants of how people feel, what illnesses they develop, and how
long they live.

YOUR RESULTS
    ATTITUDES - Misconception level   SUPPORT level
    Illness can be prevented... 1   Family................... 5
    People responsible for self 1   Friends................. 5
    Health related to feelings. 3   Community............... 4
    Habits influence longevity. 1   Place of work........... 3
    Poor health from bad luck.. 5   TOTAL (Good)............17
    Doctors do more than self.. 2
    Can reduce my health risks. 1
    TOTAL (Moderate)...........14

RECOMMENDATION
* TAKE HEALTH EDUCATION COURSE OR USE SELF-HELP INFORMATION TO GAIN POSITIVE
ATTITUDE ABOUT LIFESTYLE CHANGE, SELF RESPONSIBILITY
* SEEK SUPPORTIVE PEOPLE/GROUP WHEN MAKING LIFESTYLE CHANGES.

ROBERTS, JASON   LIFESTYLE INDEX   6/ 5/81

```
 M
 ――     MEDICAL  DATAMATION
 D
CORPORATION
         SOUTHWEST & HARRISON   BELLEVUE, OHIO 44811   AREA CODE 419 483-6060
```

LIFESTYLE INDEX REPORT   MARKETING

ROBERTS, JASON   Date Completed: 05-02-81
Age: 41 Male   Questionnaire: 1600 2753042
DOB: 06-01-40   Ht: 6' 1"   Wt: 220 lbs.

DIETARY

A well-balanced diet should contain about 55% carbohydrate (starches, sugars), 30% fat, and 15% protein by caloric proportions. Simple sugars such as dessert sweeteners or table sugar should make up less than 10% total calories. The diet should be low in saturated fats (from red meats, whole milk products), contain adequate fiber (whole grains, raw fruits), and be limited in calories to maintain ideal weight.

YOUR RESULTS

Average Daily Intake	Grams	Calories	% Daily Intake
Protein.................	70	280	15%
Carbohydrate			
Simple sugars.........60		240	13%
Other sugars........ 150		600	33%
Total carbohydrate....	210	840	46%
Fats...................	80	720	39%
TOTAL..............................		1840 Cal	100%

The daily caloric intake you indicated on your questionnaire is about 800 calories less than you are really consuming based on your weight and exercise level. In other words, you are eating more than you think, assuming that your weight is remaining constant. The "missing calories" in your diet are most likely in the form of fat in processed meats, oils, and fried foods.

Your dietary fat and simple sugar consumption are high and your dietary fiber is therefore probably low. This increases your risks for both cardiovascular disease and intestinal problems, including cancer.

You are about 31 lbs. over your ideal weight of 189.

RECOMMENDATIONS

* BE AWARE OF "MISSING CALORIES", PORTION SIZE, NUMBER OF SERVINGS.
* DECREASE RED MEAT, PROCESSED MEATS, FAT-CONTAINING DAIRY PRODUCTS, SALAD OILS, FRIED FOODS.
* DECREASE SUGAR-CONTAINING BAKED GOODS, DRINKS, DESSERTS.
* INCREASE VEGETABLES, WHOLE GRAIN CEREALS, RAW FRUITS.
* LIMIT CALORIC INTAKE, INCREASE EXERCISE TO ATTAIN IDEAL WEIGHT.

ROBERTS, JASON   LIFESTYLE INDEX   6/ 5/81

GLOSSARY

Aerobic exercise Exercise that increases the oxygen exchange in the body by increasing the heart rate through sustained activity. This type of exercise is designed to improve the efficiency of the heart. Examples are running, jogging, rapid walking, swimming, and dancing.

Angina or **angina pectoris** Severe spasmodic pain in the chest usually beneath the breast bone, caused by decreased blood supply to the heart muscle because of spasm or blockage (occlusion) of a coronary artery. It is frequently the major symptom of a coronary occlusion or heart attack.

Angiogram An X ray of a blood vessel. In this book it is used to refer specifically to an X ray of the coronary arteries to the heart.

Antibiotic A chemical substance, produced by microorganisms, that has the capacity to inhibit the growth of or destroy bacteria or other microorganisms. Antibiotics are used largely in the treatment of infectious diseases. Penicillin, produced by a mold, is one example.

Antiseptic A disinfectant that will inhibit the growth of microorganisms without necessarily destroying them. Examples are phenol (Lysol), boric acid, chlorine, and vinegar.

Aortocoronary bypass grafting A surgical procedure to increase the blood supply to the heart muscle by going around a blocked coronary artery. A vein is usually used for the graft, which is sewn in place from the aorta to the heart beyond the point where the coronary artery is blocked.

Aseptic The state of being free of disease-inducing organisms. Aseptic technique is used to prevent the introduction of pathological organisms, especially in surgery. Examples are washing the hands, wearing sterile gloves, and painting the skin with an antiseptic before making an incision.

Asymptomatic Free of symptoms. It may also refer to an early stage of a disease, before symptoms appear.

Atherosclerosis A type of hardening of the arteries (arteriosclerosis) in which the wall of the artery loses its elasticity and the opening (lumen) becomes smaller, owing to the deposit of plaques of cholesterol and lipoid materials beneath the lining membrane (intima). This type of pathology is seen in coronary artery disease.

Biliary colic Pain in the abdomen, usually in the midline or right upper quadrant, caused by spasm in the biliary tree of the liver. The cause is usually a gallstone in the gallbladder or in one of the smaller passages (the cystic or common duct) that empties into the intestine.

Biliary tree The bile ducts, which branch like a tree throughout the substance of the liver to collect bile that is formed in the liver cells.

Capitation A fee fixed at an equal sum per person (per head). This method of reimbursement is used in health maintenance organizations, where all individuals pay the same annual fee, irrespective of the number of visits or number or kind of service they receive. Usually the provider can keep any funds not used by the end of the year, but must continue to provide necessary services even if the fee has been used up. There is an incentive, therefore, not to perform unnecessary tests or treatments.

Cardiac Pertaining to the heart.

Cardiac arrest A condition in which the heart has stopped with cessation of all cardiac function and collapse of arterial blood flow. Arrest does not imply death; restoration of cardiac function is commonplace with appropriately administered cardiopulmonary resuscitation (CPR) instituted immediately.

Catheterization lab (cardiac) A laboratory equipped with X ray where flexible tubes can be inserted into a patient's vein or artery to visualize blood vessels (an angiogram) or a chamber of the heart.

Chemotherapy The treatment of a disease with chemicals. The term includes antibiotics but is not restricted to these substances. It is often used to refer to the toxic chemicals used in cancer therapy.

Cholangiogram X-ray pictures of the biliary tree, the vessels through which bile passes from the liver to the intestines. The procedure involves the administration of radio-opaque substances that are excreted by the liver and bile, or direct injection of a dye into the biliary tree, usually during operation.

Cholecystectomy Removal of the gallbladder by surgical means.

Common duct The largest duct of the biliary tree. The ducts (bile vessels) from the right and left lobes of the liver join to form the common duct, which empties into the intestines. This is frequently the site of obstruction of the biliary tree, when a stone passes out of the gallbladder, through the cystic duct, into the common duct.

Coronary Referring to arteries that supply the heart muscle. Informally, it refers to a coronary occlusion, the blockage of the artery that leads to myocardial infarction (defined below).

Cystoscopy Visualization of the inside of the urinary bladder by passing an instrument through the urethra (the canal through which urine is discharged).

Defibrillation Stoppage of fibrillation of the heart, usually by electric shock. Fibrillation is a condition characterized by twitching of the heart muscle rather than an effective contraction. It is usually fatal when it involves the ventricles (the largest portion of the heart), which pump blood into the aorta and arteries of the lungs.

DHHS Department of Health and Human Services, one of the departments of the executive branch of the U.S. government headed by a member of the President's Cabinet. This department was formerly called DHEW, Department of Health, Education, and Welfare.

EEG (Electroencephalogram) A graphic record of the electrical activity of the brain as recorded by the electroencephalograph.

EKG (Electrocardiogram) A graphic tracing of the electrical currents produced by contraction of the heart muscle.

Electrolytes Substances that, when dissolved in water, dissociate into positive and negative ions, and thereby conduct electricity. Informally, the term refers to those substances necessary for acid-base balance in the body; for instance, solutions containing sodium chloride or potassium chloride must be replaced intravenously when a patient cannot eat or drink.

Endocrinology The study of the physiology of the endocrine glands—the ductless glands whose secretions pass directly into the blood stream (such as the thyroid and adrenal glands).

FDA The Food and Drug Administration. An agency of the DHHS charged with the testing of food for any harmful additives and conducting clinical trials of new drugs before they are released.

Glucose tolerance test A test of pancreatic and liver function done by measuring blood sugar levels for several hours after giving a large dose of glucose on a fasting stomach. An abnormal test is seen with diabetes and other diseases.

Health The state of complete physical, mental, emotional, and social well-being, not merely the absence of disease or infirmity.

Hemostat A surgical instrument used to constrict a blood vessel to control or stop the flow of blood.

HHA (Health Hazard Appraisal) A computerized questionnaire that predicts the probability of an individual's developing a specific disease or diseases by matching elements of his or her lifestyle, called determinants, against previously identified risk factors for those diseases. The probabilities are based on tables of the frequency of these diseases in a specific population.

HMO (health maintenance organization) Usually a prepaid group practice that also owns, or has an exclusive contract with, a hospital and has an organization that administers insurance. Individuals contract for all their health care services to be provided over the period of a year by the organization, its hospital, and its closed panel of physicians, for a fixed capitation fee.

Immunotherapy Treatment of disease by the production of immunity.

Impotent Incapable of having an erection.

Intractable Difficult to alleviate or cure. Intractable angina pectoris, for instance, does not respond to the usual medications and results in severe disability.

IV (intravenous) urogram A roentgenogram of the urinary tract after the intravenous injection of an opaque medium that is rapidly excreted in the urine.

Lipids Fatlike substances, such as cholesterol and triglycerides. (Lipidemia—dissolved in the blood.)

Medical care Care provided by a physician. It involves mainly the diagnosis and treatment of disease and injury, but also includes the preservation and restoration of health.

Medical Establishment My term for the health care industry, a conglomerate of organized medicine, hospitals, pharmaceutical manufacturers, and health insurance companies.

Medical management Treatment of

a disease or condition without resorting to surgery. It can include any other modality, such as diet, drugs, and change in environment or lifestyle through behavior modification.

Myocardial infarction Death of the heart muscle owing to lack of blood supply. This is usually the result of a coronary artery occlusion but can also result from direct injury to the heart muscle; for instance, from a bullet wound or blunt trauma from a steering wheel injury.

Nephrology Study of the kidney and its diseases, usually including the entire urinary tract.

Open heart surgery Surgery on the heart that entails the use of a heart-lung machine to bypass the heart temporarily so it can be stopped, an incision made in its wall, and the inside of the heart exposed for direct access to the pathology by the surgeon.

OSHA (Occupational Safety and Health Administration) An agency of the federal government responsible for safety standards in industry to protect the health of and minimize the hazards to workers.

Palpation The act of feeling with the hand. The fingers are applied to the surface of the body with light pressure for the purpose of determining the consistency of the parts beneath in physical diagnosis.

Polyp A protruding growth from a mucous membrane; usually benign but occasionally malignant.

Primary care The level of care provided by a generalist, not requiring the knowledge of a specialist. This level of care can usually be provided on an ambulatory basis. About 80% of the episodes of illness for which patients seek the help of a physician fall within this level. Ideally, the care is provided by a physician who accepts responsibility for the patient's health over a long period of time. The new specialists in family practice—those certified by the American Board of Family Practice or who are Fellows of the American Academy of Family Practice—are trained to be competent in and restrict their practice to this level of care.

Prophylaxis The prevention of disease. Preventive treatment includes, for instance, immunization with a vaccine.

Prospective medicine That aspect of the practice of medicine that uses the HHA to identify risk factors and then eliminate them by behavioral change. It is risk factor intervention.

PSRO (Professional Standards Review Organization) An organization of physicians who review the medical necessity of care provided in the Medicare and Medicaid programs. PSROs were mandated as a utilization and quality-control mechanism by the Social Security amendments of 1972 (P.L. 92-603). They were based on the foundations for medical care established in California by county medical societies for the purpose of peer review.

Resuscitation To restore life or consciousness in one apparently dead. The term usually refers to cardiopulmonary resuscitation (CPR).

Retrograde pyelogram A roentgenogram of the kidney and ureter, especially showing the pelvis (cavity of the kidney that collects the urine), in which the contrast fluid is injected into the renal pelvis through the ureter during cystoscopy.

Revascularize To restore the blood supply by stimulating the growth of new blood vessels. This is the expected result of aortocoronary bypass grafting.

Roentgenogram A photograph made with X rays, named after Wilhelm Konrad Roentgen, a German physicist, the discoverer of X rays.

Secondary care The level of care provided by a specialist. A large percentage of this level of care is provided in community hospitals.

Septicemia The presence of bacterial toxins in the blood (blood poisoning).

Spirochete A spiral-shaped bacterium, One, Treponema pallidium, is the causative agent of syphilis.

Staphlococcus A spherical-shaped bacterium that occurs in clumps under the microscope. The cause of most common skin infections that produce pus.

Streptococcus A spherical-shaped bacterium that occurs predominantly in chains. Beta hemolytic Streptococcus is a dangerous pathogen in humans, causing strep throat.

Tertiary care The highest level of care, usually provided by superspecialists in academic medical centers (university hospitals), although intensive care units in community hospitals also provide this level of care.

Vasectomy Surgical removal of the *ductus (vas) deferens,* or a portion of it, as a sterilization procedure in the male.

Ventricular hypertrophy A thickening and enlargement of the wall of the ventricle of the heart. It results from pumping blood against an increase in pressure caused by pulmonary or systemic hypertension (high blood pressure).

Xenobiotics Substances foreign to the human system, usually in reference to industrial chemicals and toxic materials.

BIBLIOGRAPHY

PROLOGUE

Braunwald, E. "Coronary Surgery at the Crossroads." *New England Journal of Medicine* 297:663, 1977.

Buccino, R. and McIntosh, H. "Aortocoronary Bypass Grafting." *American Journal of Medicine* 66:663, 1979.

Miller, D., Hessel, E., Wintersheid, L. et al. "Current practice of Coronary Artery Bypass Surgery: Results of a National Survey." *Journal of Thoracic and Cardiovascular Surgery* 73:75, 1977.

Oberman, A., Jones, W., Riley, C. et al. "Natural History of Coronary Artery Disease." *Bulletin of the New York Academy of Medicine* 48:1109, 1972.

CHAPTER 1

Glandon, G. and Shapiro, R., eds. *Profile of Medical Practice 1980.* Chicago, IL: American Medical Association, 1980.

Hospital Statistics; 1982 Edition. Chicago, IL: American Hospital Association, 1982.

Hough, D. and Misek, G., eds. *Socioeconomic Issues of Health 1980.* Chicago, IL: American Medical Association, 1980.

Wilson, F. and Neuhauser, D. *Health Services in the United States.* Cambridge, MA: Ballinger Publishing Co., 1976.

CHAPTER 2

Freidson, E. *Profession of Medicine.* New York: Dodd, Mead & Co., 1975.

CHAPTER 3

Yearbook 1980. Chicago, IL: American College of Surgeons, 1980.

CHAPTER 5

Ainsworth, T. "The Millis Commission Report Revisited—a Commentary." *Hospital Medical Staff* 1;11:29, November 1972.

Millis, J. *The Report of the Citizens' Commission on Graduate Medical Education.* Chicago, IL: Council on Medical Education, American Medical Association, 1966.

CHAPTER 6

Feder, J. *Medicare: The Politics of Federal Hospital Insurance.* New York: D. C. Heath & Co., 1975.

CHAPTER 8

Medalie, J. *Family Medicine: Principles and Applications.* New York: Williams and Wilkins, 1978.

CHAPTER 9

Hardin, Garrett. "The Tragedy of the Commons." *Science* 162:1243, 1968.
Hiatt, Howard. "Protecting the Medical Commons; Who Is Responsible?" *New England Journal of Medicine* 293:235, 1975.

CHAPTER 10

Smits, H. "The PSRO in Perspective." *New England Journal of Medicine* 305:253, 1981.
Wennberg, J. and Gittelsohn, A. "Variations in Medical Practice Among Small Areas." *Scientific American* 246;4:120, April 1982.

CHAPTER 11

Falkson, J. *HMOs and the Politics of Health System Reform.* Chicago, IL: American Hospital Association, 1980; Bowie, MD: Robert J. Brady Co., 1980.

CHAPTER 12

Bryan, J., Isaacman, T., Pfeiffer, V., and Sunshine, J. "Competitive Strategies in the Health and Medical Marketplace of the 1980s." Summary Report: 1981 Bi-annual Educational Seminar, Airlie House, October 18-21, 1981. Harvard School of Public Health, Boston, MA, 1982.
Enthoven, A. "Consumer Choice Health Plan." *New England Journal of Medicine* 298:650 and 298:709, 1978.
Iglehart, J. "Drawing the Lines for the Debate on Competition." *New England Journal of Medicine* 305:291, 1981.
Durenberger, D. "The Principles of a Competition Advocate," in Iglehart, J., ed. *Health Affairs* 1:1, Winter 1981.
Ginsberg, P. "Medicare Vouchers and the Procompetition Strategy," Ibid.
Stockman, D. "Premises for a Medical Marketplace," Ibid.
Weinberger, C. "Can We Control Health Care Costs?" Ibid.

CHAPTER 13

Robbins, F. Foreword of Medalie, J., ed. *Family Medicine. Principles and Applications.* New York: Williams and Wilkins, 1978.

Summary Report of the Graduate Medical Education National Advisory Committee to the Secretary, Department of Health and Human Services. Vols. 1-7, Public Health Service, Hyattsville, MD, September 30, 1980.

CHAPTER 15

Physicians' Desk Reference. Oradell, NJ: Medical Economics, Inc., 1982.

CHAPTER 16

Gup, T. and Neumann, J. "The War on Cancer: First Do No Harm." *The Washington Post* 104;317:1 October 18,19,20,21, 1981.

CHAPTER 17

Bottoms, S., Rosen, M., and Sokol, R. "The increase in the Caesarean Birth Rate." *New England Journal of Medicine* 302:559, 1980.
Evrard, J. and Gold, E. "Caesarean Section and Maternal Mortality in Rhode Island: Incidence and Risk Factors 1965–1975." *Obstetrics and Gynecology* 50:594, 1977.
Francome, C. and Huntingford, P. "Births by Caesarean Section in the United States of America and in Britain." *Journal of Biosocial Sciences* 12:353, 1980.
Frigoletto, F. et al. "Avoiding Iatrogenic Prematurity." *American Journal of Obstetrics and Gynecology* 137:521, 1980.
Hospital Utilization Project, Pittsburgh, PA. Personal communication.
Mann, L. and Gallant, J. "Modern Indications for Caesarean Section." *American Journal of Obstetrics and Gynecology* 135:437, 1979.
Minkoff, H. and Schwartz, R. "The Rising Caesarean Section Rate: Can It Safely Be Resolved?" *Obstetrics and Gynecology* 56:135, 1980.
Nipe, G. "Jessie Bennett Decided to Operate on His Wife at Once." *Virginia Medicine* 106:884, 1979.
Saldana, L., Schulman, H., and Reuss, L. "Management of Pregnancy After Caesarean Section." *American Journal of Obstetrics and Gynecology* 135:555, 1979.

CHAPTER 18

Blagg, C. and Schribner, B. "Long-term Dialysis: Current Problems and Future Prospects." *American Journal of Medicine* 68:633, 1980.
De-Nour, A. and Shanan, J. "Quality of Life of Dialysis and Transplanted Patients." *Nephron* 25:117, 1980.
Dunea, G. "Maintenance Dialysis After Twenty Years." Editorial, *Journal of the American Medical Association* 244:67, 1980.
Kolata, G. "National Medical Care (NMC) Thrives Selling Dialysis." *Science* 208:379, 1980.
———. "Dialysis After Nearly a Decade." *Science* 208:473, 1980.

Lowrie, E. and Hampers, C. "The Success of Medicare's End-stage Renal Disease Program: The Case for Profits and the Private Marketplace." *New England Journal of Medicine* 305:434, 1981.

National Medical Care, Inc., Boston, MA. Second Quarterly Report, June 30, 1981.

Roberts, S., Maxwell, D., and Gross, T. "Cost-Effective Care of End-stage Renal Disease: A Billion Dollar Question." *Annals of Internal Medicine* 92:243, 1980.

CHAPTER 19

Directory of Medical Specialists. Published for the American Board of Medical Specialties by Marquis' *Who's Who*, Chicago, IL.

Thomas, Lewis. (Untitled). *Wilson Quarterly* 4:67, 1980.

Vickery, D. and Fries, J. *Take Care of Yourself; A Consumers' Guide to Medical Care.* Reading, MA: Addison Wesley, 1976.

CHAPTER 20

Cunningham, R. "Is the Independent Hospital an Endangered Species?" *Trustee* 35;4:23, 1982.

CHAPTER 21

Healthy People: The Surgeon's Report on Health Promotion and Disease Prevention. DHEW Publication #79-55071, Superintendent of Documents, U.S. Government Printing Office, Washington, D.C., 1979.

Knowles, J. "Doing Better and Feeling Worse: Health in the United States." *Daedalus* 106;1:1, Winter 1977.

CHAPTER 22

Robbins, L. and Hall, J. *How to Practice Prospective Medicine.* Indianapolis, IN: Slaymaker Enterprises, 1970.

CHAPTER 23

Breslow, Lester and Somers, Anne. "Lifetime Health Monitoring Program." *New England Journal of Medicine* 296:601, 1977.

Hall, J. Personal communication re study at Methodist Hospital, Indianapolis of *Diagnosis* 1980, Oradell, NJ: Medical Economics, Inc., 1980.

Terris, Milton. Editorial, *Journal of Public Health Policy* 2:305, 1981.

CHAPTER 24

Bandura, A. "The Self System in Reciprocal Determinism." *American Psychologist* 33:344, 1978.

———. *Social Learning Theory.* Englewood Cliffs, NJ: Prentice-Hall, 1977.

Belloc, N. and Breslow, L. "Relationship of Physical Health Status and Health Practices." *Preventive Medicine* 1:409, 1972.

Breslow, L. "Risk Factor Intervention for Health Maintenance." *Science* 200:908, 1978.

————. "Prospects of Improving Health Through Reducing Risk Factors." *Preventive Medicine* 7:449, 1978.

————. "Benefits and Limitations of Health Monitoring." *American Journal of Medicine* 67:919, 1979.

———— and Estrom, J. "Persistence of Health Habits and Their Relationship to Mortality." *Preventive Medicine* 9:469, 1980.

Fredrickson, D. *Harrison's Principles of Internal Medicine*, 8th ed., pp. 1297–1303. New York: McGraw-Hill, 1977.

Hammond, E. C. "Smoking in Relation to Death Rates of One Million Men and Women." National Cancer Institute Monograph 19, pp. 127-204. Department of Health and Human Services, Washington, D.C., 1966.

Farquhar, J. *The American Way of Life Need Not Be Dangerous to Your Health.* New York: W. W. Norton & Co., 1978.

The Smoking Digest; Progress Report of a Nation Kicking the Habit. Bethesda, MD: DHHS, National Cancer Institute, 1977.

Surgeon General's Report on Smoking and Health: Health Consequences of Smoking 1964, 1979. Rockville, MD: DHHS, 1981.

CHAPTER 25

Ardell, D. *High-Level Wellness.* Emmaus, PA: Rodale Press, 1977.

Selye, H. *Stress Without Distress*, New York: J. B. Lippincott, 1974.

Environmental Contaminants in Food. Congress of the United States, Office of Technology Assessment (Stock #052-003-00724-0), U.S. Government Printing Office, Washington, D.C., 1979.

CHAPTER 26

Gonnella, Joseph. "The Impact of Early Specialization on the Clinical Competence of Residents." *New England Journal of Medicine* 306:275, 1982.

Acknowledgments

A FEW WORDS of appreciation are in order for those who helped make this book a reality. Most of all I wish to thank Lila Karpf, my agent, who believed in the book from its first proposal. Special kudos are due my fellow members of the Monterey Peninsula Wednesday Night Irregulars, a group of writers who patiently listened to and criticized the many drafts of each chapter as they came from my typewriter—Joan and Tom Condon, Mary Krainik, Helen Parker, Evelyn Smart, and our mentors, Beverly Cleary and Raylyn Moore.

Ted Berry, M.D., my personal physician, author, and internist extraordinaire of Bryn Mawr, Pennsylvania and Charles Huff, M.D., my friend and Professor of Family Practice at the University of Wyoming in Casper, both offered excellent advice on the professional aspects of the text. And I sincerely appreciate the opportunity to have used the facilities and services of the Lane Medical Library of the Stanford University Medical Center for my research.

Finally, my thanks to my editor, Marion Wheeler; her assistant, Lindley Boegehold; and the staff at Macmillan who turned a rough manuscript into a book.

T.H.A.

Carmel Valley, California
November 1982

Index

Butazolidin, 117
Bypass surgery, 3–7, 115, 168, 169

Caesarean sections, 118, 125–136
Calcium, 212
Califano, Joseph, 95
Cancer, 21, 78, 114, 117, 121–122,
    140, 146, 168, 169, 176, 192,
    217, 218
  behavioral risk factors, 182, 183
  breast, 116, 179, 186
  chemotherapy, 38, 39, 63, 118,
    119–124
  hereditary factors, 180–181
  lung, 115, 119, 169, 174, 175, 179,
    183, 186–188, 192–194, 200–
    201, 219
  stomach, 119
  surgery, 120, 121
Capitation reimbursement, 164–166,
    169
Carbohydrates, 212–213
Carbon monoxide, 189
Cardiac massage, external, 2, 148
Cardiac surgeons, 2–7
Cardiologists, 60, 103n, 106, 218
  pediatric, 166
Cardiopulmonary resuscitation, 75,
    148, 155
Carmichael, Lynn, 106–107
Case-rate payment basis, 162–163, 169
Catheterization, 6, 60
Causes of disease, 180–195
Center for Disease Control, Bureau of
    Health Education, 176, 195
Cerebrovascular disease, 194
Cervical cancer, 186, 192
Charity care, 92, 99, 160
Charity Hospital, New Orleans, 57
Chemical pollutants, 181
Chemotherapy, 38, 39, 118, 120–124
Chests x-rays, 146
Childbirth, 125–136
  breech presentations, 69–70, 129,
    131–132, 135
  Caesarean sections, 118, 125–136
Chiropractors, 17, 19, 20, 178
Chlormycetin, 117
Cholangiograms, 37
Cholesterol, 168, 190, 199
  diet and, 5, 178, 211–212, 227
  risk factor intervention and, 189,
    199–201, 218, 228

testing level of, 146, 191, 193
Chronic diseases, 16, 114, 168–169,
    184–185, 188, 217–218
  See also individual diseases
Cirrhosis, liver, 176, 193, 194, 217
Clinical psychologists, licensing, 21
Clinics, 12–13, 87
Colon, cancer of, 186, 192
"Common pasture" analogy, 76–79
Community hospitals, 31, 57
Competition, 96, 97–98, 161
Comprehensive Health Manpower
    Training Act of 1971, 65
Comprehensive Health Planning Act,
    73
Computers, medical use of, 41, 116
Consumers Choice Health Plans, 96,
    160
Contraceptives, 62, 117
Cook County Hospital, Chicago, 57
Cooperatives, health care, 35
Coronary artery disease, 193
Coronary bypass surgery, 3–7, 168, 169
Coronary heart disease, 2–6, 115, 178,
    180, 197, 201, 209
Corporate practice, 36, 91
Cost reimbursement, 160, 162, 169
Council on Medical Education, 20, 43
Craniotomy, 127, 128
Crosby, Edwin, 85
Cunningham, Robert, 170

Dairy products, 212
Daly, Richard, 148
Death, 154–157
Defensive medicine, 79, 96
Dental checkups, 191, 192, 194
DeVita, Vincent, 121
Diabetes, 130, 176, 180, 200, 217
  asymptomatic, 146, 147, 186, 192,
    193
  insulin and, 62, 154
Diagnostically related diseases, 163
Diagnostic errors, 15
Dialysis. *See* Kidney disease
Diet, 4, 5, 16, 178, 211–212, 227
Diethylstilbestrol (DES), 117
Directory of Medical Specialists, 145
Disability, 138, 176
Distribution of physicians. *See*
    Physicians
Dole, Robert, 21
Drug addiction, 218